Defeating Junk Food Addiction: A $150 Billion Epidemic

(How Wellness Beat My Addiction and Help Me Lose 200 Pounds)

Brian Schneider, PhD
junkfoodaddictionandweightloss.com

There is an epidemic in America. Millions of Americans are in pain, detest the way they look and feel and believe that wellness and achieving ideal weight are goals they will never achieve. I know their frustration very well, because I was fat the better part of 40 years and never believed, with any real conviction, that I could actually lose 200 pounds, look and feel terrific and discover the keys that led to wellness and has evaded Americans for so long. But it happened. Over four years later, I'm sitting in front of my computer to tell you the events that helped changed my life forever. Your life can change too.

Every conceivable lifestyle choice: marriage, parenting, work, health and financial decisions are adversely affected by an insidious, complex and highly destructive addiction that compels Americans to spend over $150 billion annually. This addiction may often lead to loss of marriages and jobs, bouts of anxiety, depression and even death.

America is the most prosperous nation in the world, but money is simply not the solution for this addiction and it never has been. We have so much in this country and yet we are so unhealthy and ultimately living the equivalent of a time bomb lifestyle that often explodes when we least expect it to. It did for me and I'm here to tell you today that you don't have to merely exist, but you can enjoy wellness and prosperity if you want to.

Obesity is killing Americans. It is destroying our health care system. Our children are fat and unhealthy, diabetes is growing at an alarming rate and expensive weight loss programs are littering the nation to cash in on this killer epidemic. Sadly, most people don't even recognize obesity as an addiction, but they quickly accept alcoholism and drug addiction as predictable side effects of an affluent nation. Treatment is now widely accepted as a standard solution for addiction, but in truth, treatment is often not enough. Obesity is the proverbial run away train that is picking up steam and is completely out of control, destroying American's lives, yet attacking with a whisper and not a bang. It is the equivalent of opening the door for the thief to steal you blind and help him take everything you own. We are actually endorsing this tragic lifestyle and rather than expressing outrage, we simply buy more unhealthy food.

Obesity is now clearly a worldwide problem with an estimated 1.8 billion people in the world now seriously overweight. It is not just an American problem associated with affluence and privilege. It is difficult living in a prosperous society and resisting, even despising, the many creature comforts afforded us by money, technology and military dominance. Most Americans simply have no idea what life would be like if it included starvation, submission to a hostile government or to simply live a meaningless life lacking bare necessities to survive in a cold, inhumane world. We have no idea what it's like to live in obscure poverty.

However, money and advantages of a prosperous society can leave us empty and devoid of true happiness and a fulfilling life. America is a rich example of financial privilege but a nation comprised of many health problems including diabetes, cancer and cardiovascular issues due to poor lifestyle choices. The "pill for an ill" mentality that has dominated American medicine for over 80 years is accentuated by the fact that America is home to only 5% of the world's population, yet we take over 50% of the medicine prescribed today. It would be one thing if we were more healthy and productive than other nations, but we are declining in every area and our medical community is simply keeping us alive with many unpleasant operations and medicines, rather than helping us become healthy and happier. Wellness is a concept whose time has come. The medical industry is slowly converting from traditional medicine to healthy functional medical practices which are choices that most Americans generally prefer.

The Path to Prosperity

After a shocking and miserable period in my life when I gained over 100 pounds, I experienced major debt, divorce, job and financial loss, several thousand dollars in legal fees to fight a completely unnecessary battle, severe depression, anxiety and a hemorrhagic stroke that should have killed me. I survived and woke up one day to find a book that I had virtually written off for several years. This amazing book, "The Dynamic Laws of Prosperity" was written beginning in 1958 and was updated in 1995 to explain how miraculous the author's (Catherine Ponder) life was and how she survived everything from intense poverty, the death of two husbands, the trial of being a single parent and bitter loneliness and despair to achieve incredible prosperity. I can relate to her testimony and I feel my life, much like Catherine Ponder's, is a miracle and you too can enjoy wellness and prosperity .
Obesity does not have to be a life sentence and true health can be yours, perhaps for the first time in your life. Wellness is a gift and I'm convinced our Creator wants us to be well and thin, not fat and miserable, as so many Americans are today.

I believe we have a loving Creator who will help you recover lost, painful years, restore your health, finances and relationships and lead you to a fulfilling life with great joy, peace and rich prosperity. If it happened to me, it can happen to you. You must be willing to give your time, treasure or talent to get what you want in life. It is an active process, not a passive one. Catherine Ponder stated that in this initial and vital phase of prosperity, it is imperative that you will attract what you radiate. If you are radiating failure, obesity, frustration and unhappiness that is exactly what you will continue to attract. You can't get something for nothing. If you want to be thin, well and prosperous, you must start believing it and radiating that persona and that is ultimately what you will attract. It begins with faith and belief in yourself and the possibility that you will be more prosperous than you ever thought you could be. That is what our Creator wants. Life is not a short stay on the planet for a few years characterized by junk food, unsatisfactory relationships and financial misery that includes debt, privation and limited opportunities.

Prosperity, wellness, success and being thin are all processes and success always begins with the mind first. It requires "letting go" and ridding yourself of bad memories, failures, miscalculations, mistakes and exploitation. You don't want to lose weight, then gain wellness and prosperity just to have it slip away. In fact, you know from previous experiences you haven't been successful anyway, but you never understood exactly why and it has manifested as failure and low self esteem.

It is difficult to add before you subtract. You are probably saddled with countless bags of emotional trash and unfulfilled dreams that have piled up over the years and they have become so pervasive that you are literally handcuffed and paralyzed to the point you can no longer successfully function or progress and develop. Good! It's time for a change. It begins with confronting the skeletons in your closet, challenging the status quo and asserting your supreme desire for truth, peace, prosperity and wellness. It's time to lighten up.

I found it easier to begin the cleansing process on a physical level. You can begin by cleaning your car, attic, clothes drawers, garage, and any other area you may find unnecessary, old and rarely used items. Essentially, throw out any thing you can possibly live without, no longer need or would rather someone else have because your goal is what Catherine Ponder described as creating a vacuum by discarding everything you no longer want or need so you make room for the good you really want. You will experience relief and feel much more optimistic. You have made the first step in putting yourself in charge of your life and you have organized and simplified your physical existence.

Next is your emotional well being. Much like the "spring cleaning" you just experienced, take that same approach to the "mental skeletons in your mental closet" and begin a cleansing process.

This will take longer and certainly be more difficult. You must utilize a safe place and recount every dysfunctional, painful, unpleasant or problematic thought you can remember. Begin at your earliest memory and write down significant events in your life in a journal. Focus on events in school, childhood events, family affairs, friends, church, sports, hobbies and any other events or people from your childhood that you feel may be of consequence. After you've completed your journal, connect with your higher power so you might begin to understand and process or let go of any stubborn or painful negative event in your life. Ask for forgiveness for yourself or anyone else from your past so you can harmonize, stabilize and then abandon the dead past and begin making today a meaningful day. The dead past and unborn future has no place in your prosperous world.

My Junk Food Addiction Story

I began treating drug and alcohol addicts over 20 years ago. I never thought I'd see myself, some years later, struggling and grasping for understanding and an explanation of how my life could have taken so many unexplainable and painful twists that resulted in financial, marital and health challenges. I was able to achieve 3 college degrees, manage an organization that spanned 4 counties and employed 31 professionals, and endure my company closing because we were too successful and I just couldn't navigate the political waters of government billing.

I actually came to Florida in 1982 to become a National Public Radio Station Manager and taught broadcasting classes. I had just served in the Air Force almost 6 years in the American Forces Radio and Television Service. I absolutely loved broadcasting and never wanted to do anything else. It was a bitter blow leaving the station. The only consolation was the President of the college was shortly forced into retirement after I hired an attorney and showed the community how unfair he was. But I would go on to face 2 more bitter and very unfair employment experiences, which led to an undesired divorce and finally to poverty and a serious stroke that should have killed me. The nightmare didn't end there as my son was picked to help me through rehabilitation and became very resentful. He grew up and he also grew very angry and bitter.

I was forced to understand why so many Americans, like me, struggled with weight control and poor health. No one and I mean no one knew how to help me. Buying unhealthy "diet foods" sold to me by unqualified and unhealthy individuals who were essentially "sales people" was terribly disconcerting. Could you imagine if I was suffering from another addiction, such as alcohol or drugs? What an incredible disappointment.

That's what led me to form my own practice to help people just like me. It is the result of passion, hope and huge need. According to experts, 1.8 billion people in the world are **fat.** Americans spend over 150 billion dollars annually on weight control related services, food and promotion. It is by far the most insidious and common addiction in America. Yet, it is the least understood least respected and most problematic addiction in this country. Even children today are victimized by advertising and junk food availability and have so little knowledge and understanding of what is essentially a "silent addiction" that is destroying our nation by promoting divorce and family problems, employment problems, poor health and even self esteem issues. After all, who can really love and appreciate oneself when the person staring at you in the mirror is a stranger you don't want to know. Obesity is a huge problem and getting worse, especially with children. Something has to be done and that is what led me to writing this book, sharing my life with you and creating a Wellness Center to impart the knowledge I discovered to help you know the joy of being thin and well. It's what our Creator intended and how you will want to live your life. There is simply no comparison to true wellness and the Standard American Diet (SAD) and an unhealthy lifestyle. It's not a lifestyle our Creator ever intended us to live.

American health care is rapidly changing and the pressure for a more affordable and functional system continues to escalate. Our medical community continues to keep Americans alive with many unpleasant medicines and surgeries with no appreciable change. It is not entirely their fault. We have to become our own doctors and seek out functional doctors that truly appreciate and understand wellness. Most critical care doctors (the most common) should be viewed as firemen. We appreciate them willing to help us with emergencies, often at very inconvenient times, but how many visits have you made to the fire station? I thought so. We look out for ourselves and we have to look out for our health as well and we can. Our doctor should be an advisor who listens to us, understands us and is focused on wellness.

There is a loud cry in America to join the rest of the world and truly offer national health care. Wellness and functional health care are the only solutions.

Junk food addiction is the silent addiction that is so pervasive and destructive. It is America's largest and most expensive addiction. Most Americans do not consider obesity and the dysfunctional Standard American Diet as truly addictive. It is a form of denial that ironically fuels the fires for addiction, such as marketing, food manufacturer profits and fast food mentality. Junk food is fun, reasonably cheap and everywhere. And it is making us fat, sick and extremely unhealthy.

The Standard American Diet (SAD) is predicated upon and largely influenced by our visceral senses (smell, sight and taste). Most of us lack the proper knowledge to eat healthfully or we simply make bad choices dictated by our senses. In other words, we eat what we want to eat whenever our smell, taste and sight senses want to eat. They control our diet and lifestyle and they are killing us, or at least wounding us.

The average person eats about 1000 meals per year. Try an experiment. Take your age x 1000 and that's approximately how many meals you've eaten during your lifetime. The sad fact is that many Americans (some estimate over 30%) never eat digestive enzymes. Enzymes come only from raw foods such as fruits or vegetables that have never been in temperatures exceeding 118 degrees. If you are one of those persons, you're body, primarily your pancreas, must manufacture enzymes. Read the section on enzymes and see what you're missing. You need enzymes to properly assimilate food and obtain the necessary nutrients for good health. What happens if you're not one of the 30% who never gets enzymes, but you only occasionally eat enzymes? If you're 40 years old, for instance, and have eaten 40,000 meals, but only a small portion of those meals in your lifetime included digestive enzymes, you are still at risk for many health problems because you're still quite deficient. This is also how many Americans age much too rapidly and gain weight much too easily. Digestion without enzymes is very stressful and often leads to serious health problems.

Junk food addiction is a pervasive and debilitating disorder that nearly took my life and is slowly destroying America. I have over4 years clean and I will tell you I will never look back. It is so freeing to confess the truth, slay the dragon of addiction and be well. You can be well too if you want to. You'll never regret it!

Slaves to Modern Food Manufacturing

We live in a highly industrialized world driven by billions of dollars of profit and we have become slaves manipulated by the enticement of very large profits. We are inundated by so many well designed and highly destructive advertisements that we often buy unhealthy foods and consume artificial and highly toxic ingredients.

Even with the well researched and well supported information that is brought to us by medical doctors like Carolyn Dean , Russell Blaylock, Steven Sinatra and Jacob Teitelbaum, the food manufacturers continue to poison us with excitotoxins, MSG, Aspartame and other artificial and harmful additives that make us unhealthy, fat and out of control with blood sugar problems, toxic and congested livers and poor metabolism so we often end up "wearing" the food we buy because weight gain is so easy and even predictable.

We Are the Bulls Seeing Red

What we don't realize is that many food manufacturers and junk food peddlers spend a great deal of money to understand how we think, behave and what will ultimately motivate us to spend our hard earned dollars on food we don't need. It is a dangerous game and we are the bulls seeing the red flag waved at us to stimulate action which often results in careless and impractical spending habits that fuels our junk food addiction.

During a national television program recently, it was announced that most of us are stimulated or called to action by the colors red, yellow and orange. Ever wonder why school buses are painted yellow? Have you noticed that many of the manufacturers of junk food products use those colors in their packaging? Even more concerning, white has been proven to have the same effect as cocaine and it may be why so many people are attracted to flour and sugar. Junk food addiction and other kinds of addiction are closely related because stimuli such as colors can trigger the brain to respond and just as bulls react to red without caution, we respond and eat food that we know isn't healthy, but have little remorse. The greedy junk food pushers are feeding our junk food addiction and virtually no one is paying attention. Its why so many of us are like zombies lined up for junk food and associate it with American culture. It tastes good, so it must be good. Junk food is addictive and "one drink will kill you" is how alcoholics and drug addicts are able to stay clean and control their addiction. We don't need junk food and there are plenty of viable options and I guarantee you if the food manufacturers knew they couldn't poison us; they would produce many satisfying and healthy alternatives. It's up to us.

Many of the ingredients used by manufacturers stimulate our appetite, are virtually irresistible and lead to us buying more of it and ultimately succumbing to a lifelong junk food addiction which may lead to metabolic syndrome, blood sugar problems, toxic liver, hypothyroidism, cardiovascular problems and obesity.

It is a vicious cycle and this book is dedicated to all the victims (like you and me) who have been manipulated and used by greedy and ruthless food manufacturers, fast food companies and junk food pushers who have managed to legally and without so much as a whisper from us, manipulate and use us to fatten their wallets. Look at all the obese kids, the national epidemic of diabetes, the increasing rate of cancer and cardiovascular patients and the alarming rate of obesity in America today. It is America's worst, most destructive and most expensive addiction and we don't even admit it's an addiction. It's time to discover wellness for you and your loved ones. It is our only hope.

The Cause of Junk Food Addiction

When we examine alcoholism and drug addiction, often biological or hereditary factors are mentioned as specific reasons that lead to these destructive syndromes. Sometimes nutritional deficiencies are cited as causes for supporting or perpetuating both addictions. Of course lifestyle factors centered on bad decisions, mistakes, poor choices, negative events and destructive friendships support or may lead to alcoholism and drug addiction. For many, it becomes a lifestyle and addiction is a lifelong process. Even AA and NA meetings are typically associated with caffeine (coffee), cigarettes and junk food addiction. It can be a lifelong process and a self-induced jail sentence with decisions and lifestyle choices made with their addiction as a guiding or determining factor.

Junk food addiction is the most prevalent addiction in our country, yet it is virtually undetected, unnoticed and untreated. The primary etiology or cause of junk food addiction is not closely related to the other addictions of alcoholism, tobacco addiction and drug addiction. The main factor that causes junk food addiction is hedonism or pleasure seeking. In a nation dominated by external pleasure, we are programmed from birth to seek pleasure and essentially convert everything we approach into a pleasurable scenario so that we will enjoy and not endure it as hardship. This from a nation of people with short attention spans, unhealthy physiques, dominated by the media and spoiled by a powerful military that has managed to keep us safe and relatively unscathed.

Our hedonism has caused our school and work performance to suffer, to spend money on entertainment, junk food and lavish abundance. Hedonism has caused and perpetuated divorce and ultimately led to very unhealthy lifestyles. Only 10% of Americans exercise, we take most of the world's medicines, more people are divorced than married today and our kids are now being raised in a very complex and dysfunctional society. Hedonism is the root of our junk food addiction and it feeds the serious problems that typify American behavior.

We honestly believe we can continue to live unhealthy, unstable and dysfunctional lives that will somehow be managed or fixed by government, medicine or counseling. They won't though. Our problems will only become worse.

Instead of seeking pleasure, why not seek harmony, knowledge, peace, wellness, love and ultimately prosperity, which is the healthy combination of all of them. We have essentially sought hedonism since World War II, a time when this country came together to fight evil around the world and unified in harmony as we became the greatest nation on earth. Since that time, hedonism has been the major religion in this country and junk food is the diet that has fueled it. It is a vicious merry-go-round that is now on auto-pilot. Advertising, food manufacturers and drug manufacturers are all profiting from our largest addiction. Children have been indoctrinated in junk food addiction and have now accepted it as a way of life.

We have seen cigarette smoking decrease, treatment centers are now common and plentiful for drug addiction and alcoholism, but our nation's largest and most expensive addiction – junk food addiction – marches on silently taking prisoners while enjoying widespread acceptance or passive rejection. It is a stealth assassin and is virtually indestructible. It is a predictable disease associated with an affluent society, but just as we have admitted and are now treating the other addictions that have caused so much pain, we must recognize junk food addiction, treat hedonism and pursue wellness. Functional medicine, better food labels, more healthy foods, better food growing and manufacturing laws, better school lunches and strong promotion of wellness is the answer to treating our nation's largest and most expensive addiction. It is time to recognize, treat and eliminate junk food addiction and seek prosperity. The future is now.

The Wellness Model

A. All disease is primarily based on (3) different events
        1. Oxidative Stress
        2. Toxic Buildup
        3. Acidic pH

1. **Oxidative Stress** - Free radical damage is also known as oxidative stress. Free radicals are unstable molecules (meaning they have an unpaired electron) produced within our bodies. Free radicals damage healthy cells by "stealing" an electron from the healthy cell in order to become stable. Free radicals are naturally occurring molecules present in every person. However, internal and external factors such as diet, lifestyle, activity levels, chemicals and

pollutants can increase the levels of free radicals, and thereby increase the risk of damage from free radicals. Oxidative stress can be minimized by a supplement called **Protandim (theultimatepill.net)**. Taking this supplement daily will increase your body's natural antioxidant system and has been proven (with aldehyde testing) to lower your oxidative stress level 40% within 30 days to the level of a 20 year old.

2. **Toxic Buildup** - As a result of internal and external factors, such as the Standard American Diet (SAD), a sedentary activity level, stress, chemicals, pollutants and other factors, our bodies produce toxins. A toxic build

up occurs and, especially as we age, the toxins will normally lead to illness, premature aging and even death. When we detoxify, we may experience unpleasant symptoms, such as fogginess, lethargy, irritability, confusion, aches and pains and general malaise. This process is known as the Herxheimer Effect. Many people will prematurely cease or fail with detoxification because of the unpleasant side effects associated with die-off of toxins known as the Herxheimer Effect. Choosing **FIR (Far Infrared therapy),** which utilizes sweat as a detoxification channel, is a very good modality to minimize and usually eliminate all side effects.

3. **Acidic pH** – Otto Warburg, M.D. received the Nobel Prize award for his ground-breaking work asserting that no disease can thrive in an alkaline environment. Most Americans have a total body pH that is below 7.0 and is considered acidic. Our blood is always alkaline (measuring 7.4 pH) and any slight variation can be very harmful, even fatal. Our total body pH should also be slightly alkaline. Many cancer and other seriously ill patients have very acidic pH levels which confirms Warburg's assertion. Many strategies, including drinking alkaline water and eating a whole foods organic diet, primarily

vegetarian, along with a water ionizer such as **Rejuvenator (watershed.net)** detoxify your body of acidic waste and are very helpful in achieving an alkaline pH.

Metabolic Weight Loss Program Benefits

1. Body Fat Percentage Reduction
2. Blood Sugar Balance
3. Appetite Control
4. Energy Increase
5. Hormonal Balance
6. Cardiovascular Improvement
7. Lowered Cholesterol
8. Lowered Triglycerides
9. Increased Antioxidants
10. Increased Digestive Enzymes
11. Immune Function Improvement
12. Liver Decongestion
13. Improved Digestion
14. Reduced Inflammation
15. Disease Prevention
16. Scale (weight) Loss
17. Increased pH (alkalinity)
18. Improved Hydration
19. Lowered Free Radicals
20. Reduced Toxic Load

How to Detoxify in 5 Easy Steps

This Program will help you:
- *Lose Weight*
- *Have More Energy*
- *Have Better Bowel Movements*
- *Lower Cholesterol*
- *Lower Blood Pressure*
- *Improve Hair, Skin and Nails*

Step 1

Take DE (1 tablespoon daily)

Step 2

Drink Ionized Water (Rejuvenator)

Step 3

Eliminate almost 300 sextillion free radicals daily (Protandim)

Step 4

Rub Magnesium Oil on your body every night

Step 5

Use an FIR sauna 30 minutes daily

Step 1 -Detoxification with Diatomaceous Earth

One of the major obstacles with treating any illness, particularly weight gain, is the dilemma of a toxic body and all the complications it presents. When a person possesses a coated colon and a body full of toxins, any medicine or natural substance used to treat a problem will be often be ineffective.

According to **earthworkshealth.com**, there are 3 major ways in which a product that I have used with many clients, called **Diatomaceous Earth** (Food Grade), works to detoxify the body and rid it of the harmful elements that often sideline or even cause a weight loss program to fail.

Diatomaceous Earth – when magnified 7000 times - looks like a cylinder full of holes--kind of like Rice Chex Cereal. This cylinder has a very strong negative charge. As these millions of cylinders move through the stomach and digestive tract, they attract and absorb fungi, protozoa, viruses, endotoxins, pesticides and drug residues, E-Coli, and heavy metals. These are trapped inside the cylinder and passed out of the body. In addition, any larger parasites that happen to be in the stomach or digestive tract are "cut up" and killed by the sharp edges of the Diatomaceous Earth. All of these activities result in a much healthier body with less sickness. People often say "I just feel better" with Diatomaceous Earth. This better feeling comes from all the "junk" being removed from the body and by giving the immune system the "jump start" it needs.

2nd

Diatomaceous Earth is **very** hard. On the hardness scale where diamonds are a 9, Diatomaceous Earth is a 7. This is very important, because as those millions of tiny hard and sharp Diatomaceous Earth cylinders pass through the small and large intestines, they "scrub" the walls. After only a few months of taking Diatomaceous Earth, the intestine wall is no longer coated with mucus and molds but CLEAN!! The advantages of this are several:

1. Regular bowel movements (This is the #1 comment everyone makes about DE)
2. Healthier Colon. This is especially important as we get older. A clean healthy colon keeps away polyps, cancers, and ulcers. Today, many are spending thousands of dollars to get colonics to do the same thing as Diatomaceous Earth does.
3. Many users report increased energy and needing less sleep. This is a result of all the food and nutrients that are taken in being better absorbed into the blood stream. With a coated colon--many nutrients never get absorbed.

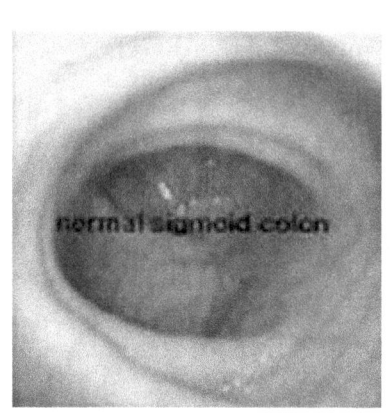

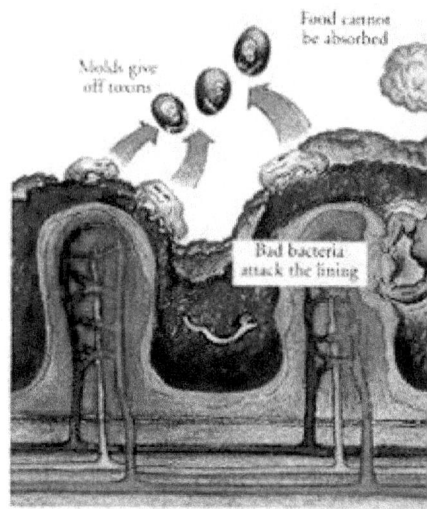

3rd

A small amount of Diatomaceous Earth gets absorbed into the blood stream as silica. One of the benefits of Silica is that it helps to destroy bad fats. Most people taking Diatomaceous Earth have lowered their cholesterol by 40-50 points. They are also amazed at how their high blood pressure goes down.

1. Sore joints and ligaments feel better
2. Skin clears up (acne-age spots-psoriasis)
3. Hair and nails are stronger and grow faster
4. Stronger teeth and gums
5. Healthier respiratory tract--less coughing
6. Menopause has less symptoms
7. Healthier urinary tract

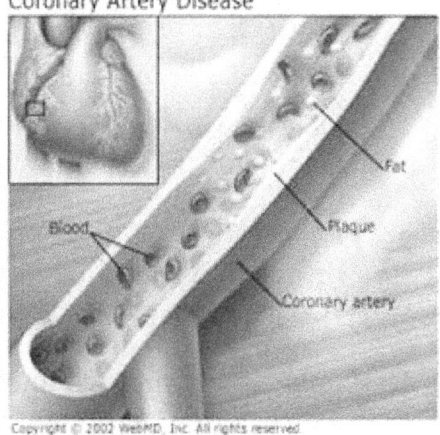
Coronary Artery Disease

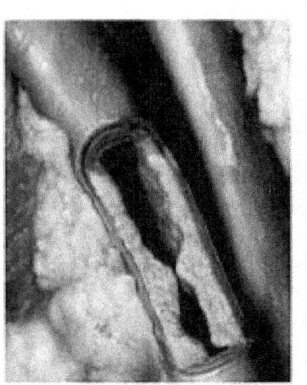

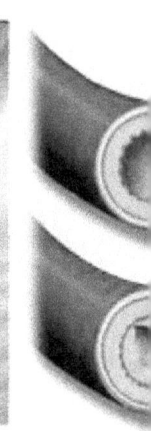

The benefits of silica are many. In today's grains, there is actually a shortage of silica. Years ago, the silica found in our foodstuffs was adequate, but with today's hybrids and depleted soils, only about 1/3 of the silica needed is supplied in our food. Diatomaceous Earth is a simple and inexpensive way to get the silica your body needs.

I have tried many detoxification programs over the years, but I have never tried anything as easy and effective as Diatomaceous Earth. It really works!

Step 2 – Drink Ionized Alkaline Water

Obesity is actually protecting our bodies and acts as insulation to the highly acidic lifestyle we lead. Ionic water can literally save our lives and end (for many of us) a lifelong obesity problem. I recommend **Rejuvenator Ionizer (<u>watershed.net</u>).** Rejuvenator is the world's smallest water ionizer and costs only $40 (compared to many water machines over $4000). If you let Rejuvenator sit in the water for at least 5 minutes, your water should be close to 9.0 pH. If you eat healthy, alkaline foods, your total body pH should be near 7.4 (the same as your blood). Otto Warburg, MD won the Nobel Prize in 1931 because he proved that when our bodies become alkaline (over 7.0 pH), no disease can survive in an alkaline environment.

The term alkaline water is just a label used to describe ideal drinking water as provided by nature; one of many labels that arise as we explore the hidden properties of water. **Alkaline water has more excess oxygen and alkaline minerals than neutral or acid tap water**. It is highly oxygenated water with the oxygen form that is needed by our cells. Alkaline water has 100's of times more excess oxygen then neutral tap water and no acid elements or toxic substances in it. The discovery of ionized water closely replicates the living qualities of high altitude mountain spring water: Fresh, Invigorating, Life Enhancing, Free Radical Scavenging and Delicious.

Alkaline water is drinking water as it should be, and as it is in nature's best waters like glacier waters. If you measure the properties of glacier water, considered the very best drinking water, it has similar properties to ionized water - alkaline pH, high colloidal mineral content, active hydrogen and micro clusters. In nature you see a separation of water into acid and alkaline: high altitude spring waters tend to be alkaline (for drinking), whereas hot spring waters are acidic (but have a reputation for skin cleansing). .

Ionized alkaline and acid waters are used in hospitals and clinics throughout Japan and South Korea, where the water ionizer is classified as a medical device.

Ionized water is considered to be one of the most effective and easy ways for your body to: hydrate, alkalize and detoxify. Alkaline water can **slowly reverse the aging process,** which is a gradual process of acid waste accumulation. It is every effective because the water penetrates deeply to dissolve and remove toxins from the body. Acid wastes like lactic acid that are insoluble in neutral water become soluble in alkaline water and so can be removed from the body by drinking alkaline water. Alkaline water has many reported benefits. It can help with **weight loss**, help the body detoxify, reduce the aging process, help in cases of diabetics and other health conditions, provide valuable anti-oxidants, and help prevent cancer.

Slightly alkaline blood pH ensures that micro-organisms remain in harmony with the body. When the pH becomes acidic there is a lack of oxygen which causes a proliferation of antagonistic, anaerobic microforms to appear. The acidic body becomes a breeding ground for germs, fungus and viruses. They consume the food we eat and leave us more acid waste excrements! Acidity coagulates blood and clogs up the capillaries. Over-acidity interferes with life itself, leading to virtually all sickness and disease including heart attacks and cancer, premature aging and **obesity.**

Our 75 trillion cells are slightly acidic within and are surrounded by slightly alkaline interstitial fluid around them. This polarity is essential for chemical or energy interchange, and is lost with acidity - one reason why so many people lack energy. Acidic pH interferes with mineral absorption. We will receive no iodine unless the body pH is almost perfect and calcium is very difficult to absorb with an excessively acid body. Excess acidity weakens all our systems and forces the body to take minerals from vital organs and bones to buffer/neutralize the acid and safely remove it from the body. The body creates cholesterol (fatty deposits) to safely store deadly crystallized acid wastes away from vital organs of liver, heart and kidney. '**_Obesity is an acid problem, the fat is saving our lives_**' explains Dr Robert Young

Step 3 – Eliminate Free Radicals

What Causes Free Radicals?

Free radicals are cells that are searching for an electron and become out of control and very unpredictable. They can be destructive by accelerating the aging process, land in joints which may cause inflammation and arthritis or lead to serious diseases, such as cancer. The pollution that makes the 21st century so dangerous and complex along with consuming the Standard American Diet (SAD) consisting of junk food with artificial ingredients has led to increased inflammation and free radical activity. We live in dangerous times that require our immediate attention and action if we are to lead long, healthy lives.

Free radicals can come from our own metabolism, pollution, heavy metals, cigarette smoke, impure water, processed foods, drugs, magnesium and silica (minerals) deficiency, excitotoxins (such as Aspartame which is used to flavor diet drinks). Free radicals are simply a major part of our lifestyle and cannot be avoided.

Free Radical Elimination

Scientific studies indicate that we produce about 300 sextillion (that's 21 zeroes) free radicals every day. It is a major reason why we are becoming sicker and dying younger. Free radicals are closely associated with an affluent culture. The problem with taking antioxidants is that they eliminate free radicals on a 1 to 1 basis. You couldn't possibly take enough antioxidants to eliminate 300 sextillion free radicals daily. So what's the solution?

Protandim (ultimatepill.net) is a formula designed by a PhD who received his degree from Duke University and has been nominated for the Nobel Prize. He discovered SOD, which is a natural antioxidant enzyme in your body. Protandim activates your own antioxidant enzymes and you then eliminates 1 million free radicals per second for 24 hours when you take 1 Protandim pill which incorporates 5 herbs. Protandim is an easy all-natural way to eliminate a major problem so you can have more energy, prevent many diseases and lead a healthy life.

Step 4 - The Miracle of Magnesium

1. Helps to lower cholesterol
2. **Magnesium can help prevent obesity**
3. Great for insomnia and sleep problems
4. Lowers risk of heart disease (especially hypertension)
5. Helps prevent strokes
6. Helps treat diabetes
7. Improves mood and memory

8. Helps prevent depression and anxiety
9. Effectively prevents and treats headaches and pain
10. Useful in treatment of Chronic Fatigue and Fibromyalgia

* I recommend rubbing Magnesium Oil on your body every night

Step 5 -The FIR Sauna Benefits

1. **Average weight loss** – 1 pound per week (daily 30 minute sessions)
2. **Calories expended** – 600 to 2400 calories per 30 minute session
3. **Cleansing/Detoxification** – Lymphatic and Immune System
4. **Cardiovascular Benefits** – 6 mile run per 30 minute session
5. **Improves relaxation and sleep**
6. **Facial Cleansing** (reduces toxins)

The FIR Sauna is light, portable, unzips and can be washed and hung to dry, easily transported in the trunk of a small car, arm vents allows freedom to use laptop computer, phone, watch TV or listen to music.

The FIR sauna has been endorsed by NASA (used by the astronauts), American Heart Association, used by many hospitals, health clubs all over the world and is especially effective at **burning fat.**

The Wellness Shield

1. Acai Juice – (ORAC – 1026)
2. Green Tea – (200 times more powerful than Vitamin E, increases immune function by 500%)
3. Watercress- Repairs DNA, Scored 1000 (perfect Score) on Nutrition Test
4. Broccoli, Cabbage, Cauliflower – Indole - 3 Carbinol
5. Carrots, Tomatoes – Carotenoids
6. Onions, Apples – Quercetin
7. Soy (Edamame, Miso, Tofu) – Genistein
8. Curry- Curcumin
9. D – Ribose – Increases energy by 45%, lowers blood sugar
10. Sea Salt – 25% less sodium
11. Grapeseed Oil – High Smoke Point (good for cooking)
12. Flaxseed, Coconut, Olive Oils – Healthy at room temperature

- Omega-3 (anti-inflammatory fat) – Salmon, Flaxseed, Walnut, Omega-3 eggs

Appetite Suppressing Scents
1. Banana
2. Peppermint
3. Green Apple

smellandtaste.org – Allan Hirsch, M.D.

The Wellness Numbers

1. Body Fat Percentage – (Males – 15%), (Females – 20%)
2. Blood Sugar – A1C Hemoglobin 6.0
3. Blood Pressure – 115/75
4. Total Cholesterol – 200
5. HDL Cholesterol – 60
6. LDL Cholesterol - 100
7. Triglycerides - 100
8. pH – 7.4 (after 4 hour fast)
9. Hydration – 64 ounces daily water intake (or more)
10. Aldehydes - 300 (Free Radical Breathalyzer Test)

The Digestive Process

Let's examine what happens when we eat food and review the digestion process. First, the food needs digestive enzymes when it hits the tongue. We've already talked about the pancreas. After we've chewed our food and broken it down, it can move through the digestive system. It stops at the liver, which performs over 200 functions. The liver is also the only organ in the body that can expel or get rid of your own fat. The liver, like many of your other organs, is constantly assaulted by your bad choices. Remember, that's a lifetime of meals without digestive enzymes which has probably caused you countless problems including several trips to the drug store or the doctor's office for medicine. Americans are spending billions of dollars on drugs and surgeries to cover up poor lifestyle, specifically eating, habits. The pizza tasted good, the dessert was delicious for about 5 minutes. You've heard it before.....a moment on the lips and a lifetime on the hips.

Back to the liver. If we really want to take care of your largest organ, it needs milk thistle and a liver friendly diet (as in this program). Silymarin is the active ingredient in **milk thistle** and we should take about 400 mg daily or 2000 mg of the whole milk thistle herb. Liver friendly foods, such as carrots, beets, celery, watermelons, apples and dark green vegetables will truly make our livers happy.

Moving on to the pancreas. Another organ, like the liver, that is under major assault by the Standard American Diet. The pancreas hates processed sugar and junk food. A staple or at least major part of, most people's diet. This is exactly why so many Americans become diabetics and some are now slaves to a dialysis machine which costs them $250,000 per year. The pancreas manufactures most of our digestive enzymes which are so critical to our health, yet we assault the very organ that is trying to keep us well and live longer. The pancreas can benefit by taking **alpha-lipoic acid** and **chromium picolinate**. Just like the liver, the pancreas wants whole, healthy organic food and not the junk so many Americans stuff down their throats every day. We should replace the processed sugar we eat so much with **Stevia, d-ribose, even maple syrup and buckwheat honey** are much better than processed sugar. They are real foods. The good fats (Omega 3) found in ocean **fish, Omega 3 eggs, walnuts and flaxseeds** are good for every part of your body because they are anti-inflammatory. Inflammation can be described as taking a syringe with colored fluid and putting a drop in water. The entire container will turn the color of the fluid. Omega 3 fats are anti-inflammatory and will stop the inflammation, which will lead to good health and longer life. The pro-inflammatory and processed sugar American diet is extremely difficult for the pancreas and liver. An anti-inflammatory diet specifically promotes better cardiovascular health, the #1 killer of Americans.

Not forgetting about **digestive enzymes**, our body produces over 6000 enzymes and they can protect us from arthritis, cancer and so many other degenerative diseases, not to mention those painful and annoying stomach and bowel problems. Taking digestive enzymes in your daily vitamin supplement and eating whole, natural foods that contain digestive enzymes, such as raw fruits and vegetables, will make your pancreas and liver so much more effective and ultimately lead to good weight management.

After our food leaves the pancreas, the next consideration in the digestive process is the gut. Health begins and ends in the gut. Over 70% of our immune function is controlled by the gut. If we want to truly practice wellness and maintain our weight effectively, we have to think of our gut as a lawn that needs fertilizer to feed the healthy grass and weed killer to crowd out or kill the weeds and bad plant growth. **Probiotics** acts as both. It feeds the good bacteria, such as **lactobacillus acidophilus** and eliminates the bad bacteria, such as streptococcus. It is important to use a good Probiotics that has several strains of good bacteria and at least 10 billion CFU (colony forming units).

Fiber, elimination, and bowel movements are also important to good health and can play a critical role with appetite, food choices and weight maintenance. Colon health also relies on eating enough good fiber. We need to have

40 grams of fiber daily to have the desired 1-3 daily bowel movements with toothpaste texture, not diarrhea or constipation. Most Americans eat 10 grams of fiber daily.

A good yardstick to measure the fiber you eat and ensure you're getting enough is to remember this – 1 serving of fruit or 1 whole fruit is about 3 grams, 1 serving of vegetables or 1 whole vegetable is 4 grams, and 1 serving of beans is 7 grams of fiber. Grains and nuts or seeds also have fiber and you can normally find out on the nutrition label. Typically, 1 cup equals 1 serving. Most Americans eat approximately 10 grams of fiber daily and have 1-3 bowel movements **weekly**. Again 40 grams of fiber and 1-3 bowel movements **daily** (with toothpaste consistency) is the desired amount. Getting the correct fiber and Probiotics can be very helpful with the immune system and good weight management. One more thing about the gut, it is estimated by experts that 90% of our emotional state is controlled by our gut. The chemicals in our body that control our mood (serotonin – depression, dopamine – anxiety) are affected by gut health. Some scientists call the gut our second brain and it's easy to see why. It's also an important part of a weight loss program. Many problems can be prevented with good gut health.

I believe the healthiest fiber you can eat is **Glucomannan**. It improves the liver's ability to excrete waste, lowers cholesterol, alleviates PMS symptoms such as bloating, water retention and irritability, reduces headaches, reduces hunger and controls appetite.

Leaving the gut and moving up the body, we'll stop next at the kidneys and adrenal glands. The kidneys love water and many diabetics have kidney trouble that may lead to dialysis and costs them $250,000 a year for daily treatments. You do not want to be a diabetic that needs dialysis. Is sugar really worth it? As I was saying, your kidneys love water and it's very important to drink at least a half-gallon of fresh, pure water daily. I personally drink about 3 – 32 ounce glasses every day or 96 ounces daily. Our body needs water, especially kidneys. Many people are overweight because they are dehydrated and mistake thirst for hunger. Water can also be an excellent appetite suppressor. Drinking enough water should help reduce headaches and provide more energy. Remember, caffeine found in coffee and soda causes dehydration as well. That's why it's a good idea to drink mostly water on a weight reduction program, but in general water is a great idea.

The Adrenal Glands

Like the pancreas and liver, the adrenal glands are victims of 21st century lifestyles. The Standard American Diet (SAD) and 21st century stress wreak havoc on the adrenal glands. A hormone called cortisol will be elevated when you ingest sugar and live the stressful modern life that unfortunately does not include enough sleep and exercise. Some people call Cortisol the "death hormone." Too much stress and poor diet will have an impact on the adrenal glands and will result in sleep disturbance, lower energy and poorer control of junk food, especially sodas with caffeine and foods with processed sugar. The water soluble **vitamins B and C, especially the B vitamins (1, 2, 3, 5, 6, 12 and folate or folic acid),** are critical for stress management. Both vitamins B-Complex and C are water soluble meaning it doesn't matter how much you take in the morning, by early evening (about 12 hours later) the vitamins will be gone and you will be depleted through the night. That's why a timed release version of the vitamins or taking them twice a day is necessary. The depletion of the stress and water soluble vitamins is one reason the adrenal glands are overworked and under supported. **Magnesium** is also very helpful in relaxing the whole body and managing stress. Magnesium should be taken topically as oil or crème where it can travel through the blood into the gut. You can't take too much and Dr. Carolyn Dean indicates in her book, "The Magnesium Miracle" that magnesium serves 325 enzymes in the body and relaxation and sleep are much better with magnesium. Anxiety induced sleep deprivation can also lead to poor eating habits because people will often want to compensate by eating sugar or drinking caffeine. Both foods often lead to obesity and health problems, including premature aging.

The #1 and #3 killers in this country are both cardiovascular diseases: heart attacks and strokes. The root cause of cardiovascular diseases is stress and restricted blood flow (atherosclerosis). Inflammation (from eating the bad fats and junk food) is often the cause of atherosclerosis and impaired adrenal function resulting from stress can be a deadly combination. That is why cortisol is often called the "death hormone." Many obese people, especially the "type A" personalities experience overwhelming stress and must take magnesium and B complex along with more rest, relaxation and daily exercise to combat the uncomfortable stress that often prevents them from safe and effective weight management. It is also a good idea to test for food allergies or food sensitivities to rule out any problems associated with diet.

Sometimes yeast or Candida can exacerbate the situation. **Oil of Oregano** and the elimination of sugar and yeast often prove to be an effective tool to combat the symptoms associated with the "leaky gut syndrome", the catalyst that may produce Candida and an overwhelming desire to eat sugar and result in weight gain. This happened to me and eventually produced Chronic Fatigue Syndrome characterized by insomnia, lethargy and weight gain. A common occurrence among "type A personalities." Again, the combination of poor diet (junk food) and stress may lead to the "leaky gut syndrome", especially American's infinity for sugar and unhealthy food. It's imperative to also eliminate processed sugar and replace it with **Stevia, d-ribose**, and low glycemic fruits that will satisfy your sweet tooth as well as

chromium picolinate and alpha-lipoic acid to balance the blood sugar. America's fascination with sugar and our enormous appetite for it have propelled us into food addiction and is slowly wounding and killing us, yet we don't view it as seriously as we do drug and alcohol addiction.

The Immune System

Most people have no idea which organs in the body belong to the immune system. The immune system consists of white blood cells, the lymphatic glands, adenoids, thymus, spleen, tonsils, the mucus membranes of the gastrointestinal (GI) system and respiratory tract. Symptoms of a problematic immune system may include colds, flu, chronic fatigue, infection and frequent illnesses. Free radicals may weaken our immune system also. Other lifestyle factors such as smoking, drinking, poor diet and lack of exercise all contribute to a weakened and ineffective immune system. Overeating, especially junk food is often the remedy of relief to escape from pain, hence the term "escape behavior". We often go to great lengths to escape from pain or undesirable consequences. Rather than choose a lifestyle focusing on wellness, we choose escape behavior that includes junk food and leads to additional, more serious problems. The "pill for an ill" has been a staple for the medical industry and pharmaceutical companies to temporarily remedy problems. The nutrients **beta glucan, olive leaf extract, royal jelly (from the bee), Colostrum and Probiotics** have all proven to be effective with many immune system disorders. The FIR sauna has an excellent track record with the immune system and is particularly effective at supporting the lymphatic gland.

The Hormonal System

The hormonal system is often functional for most males until they reach their 40's. After that age, a decline occurs and men over 50 years of age typically have lowered testosterone and DHEA levels that lead to weight gain, poor sleep habits and low energy. Regular exercise, caffeine and sugar restriction, better sleep, proper hydration and a healthy diet all become necessary for good health. This is also a good age when magnesium or **7-keto DHEA** may be a good supplementation to increase energy, concentration and improve sleep. Wellness is critical in the middle age years and poor lifestyle habits may lead to many problems, including death.

Women, however, must monitor hormone levels which can fluctuate during menses. Estrogen dominance is a common problem and may lead to PMS (premenstrual syndrome), bloating, weight gain and endometriosis. Perimenopause may increase heart disease risk up to 400%. Blood pressure levels should be checked frequently. As with men, DHEA levels typically begin to fall by the 40's and are typically low by the 50's and beyond. DHEA supplementation can be dangerous and is controversial, but 7-keto DHEA is regarded as safe and available to the public. Hormone therapy utilizing saliva testing and bioidentical hormone replacement carefully monitored by qualified physicians may be a good option. Hormone related issues, particularly for women, can be a major factor in weight management and obesity.

The Neurological System

Neurological issues, particularly diseases, such as Alzheimer's, dementia and Parkinson's are often associated with elderly, but many younger people are very concerned about one day contracting a neurological disease. Aspartame and many of the chemicals prevalent in our society today and part of our diet are known to cause neurological disorders and should be avoided. Natural, chemical free organic food is the best and safest option. Poor memory, better concentration and mental acuity are all concerns for many people. **Fish oil, gingko biloba and phosphatidlyserine** are supplements that support a healthy neurological system as well as constructive mental activity such as puzzles and games that require concentration and increased mental activity.

The Liver

Most people are totally unaware of how vitally important the liver is to our health and particularly the role it plays in obesity. It is vital to metabolism and serves over 500 functions in your body. The liver is often the main reason we will lose weight or be unsuccessful and frustrated as most of us have been. It is so hard to believe, but if we simply follow a liver-friendly diet, take the right supplements, utilize the FIR sauna, drink enough water and walk whenever you can you will have great success. At one point, I lost a pound per day and most people will lose at least 2 pounds per week, depending on how much you need to lose. The liver is the key organ involved in fat loss. It is the supreme metabolism organ and when it is not working properly and being fed liver unfriendly food as most of us do, there are typically symptoms ranging from bloating, poor digestion, fatigue, headaches, unpleasant mood, irritable bowel syndrome, sluggishness, poor immune function, excessive body heat, high cholesterol, gall bladder problems, sugar cravings, fatty liver, intolerance to alcohol, high blood pressure, allergies and an inability to lose weight. Our program includes the right nutrients, a liver friendly diet, FIR sauna to help you detoxify, drinking enough water and the right amount of walking and rest to activate your liver to help you burn fat and be well. If you are like so many people who have struggled to lose weight and stay healthy for many years to find that weight loss becomes an elusive goal always out of reach. Unwanted pounds begin to pile up and frustration mounts as medical bills become a part of your life and you begin to doubt yourself and desperation rules your life. You'll try anything, yet nothing seems to work. Am I fat for the rest of my life? Can anyone help me?

The most overlooked and misunderstood organ in the human body is the liver. It performs over **500 functions** 24 hours a day and it is by far the most overworked and one of the most mistreated organs in our body. Our livers typically become congested in our 30's and we begin to experience the consequences including weight gain, adult acne, bowel disorders, digestive complaints, low energy, headaches, depression, gall bladder problems, hypertension, blood sugar problems and many other complaints.

It is important to cleanse, repair and maintain your liver to effectively lose weight, correct most, if not all of your physical complaints and enjoy wellness. Your liver is actually capable of expelling or getting rid of your own fat. Unfortunately, many people's livers are so congested and unhealthy they actually accumulate or hold onto fat instead of expelling it. No wonder so many people are fat and unhealthy. This program will help you to detoxify your liver with the following guidelines.

1) The Meal Plan is comprised of delicious, liver-friendly foods that will support healthy liver function.

2) Supplements, such as **milk thistle**, will help detoxify, restore and revitalize your liver so it will help burn off unwanted fat and help you become well.
3) The Far Infrared Sauna will detoxify and support your liver. NASA and the American Heart Association endorse FIR saunas and many health clubs and hospitals around the world utilize FIR saunas.
4) Drink at least 64 ounces or one half gallon of water daily to flush out toxins and impurities in your liver.
5) I recommend daily movement, particularly walking, dancing, bicycle riding –anything you can do to move, stretch, build muscle and increase your heart rate is very helpful. Daily movement helps weight loss, gives you energy, excellent cardiovascular support and improves liver function.

The liver is one of the most important organs in the body, particularly regarding weight loss. Love your liver and get well today.

There are several vital principles necessary to lose weight and improve your liver function.

1) Avoid eating sugar, especially processed sugar. Instead, eat d-ribose, Stevia, low glycemic fruits, even maple syrup and honey are better choices. America's passion for sugar is destroying liver and pancreas function.

2) Avoid foods you are allergic to. Get a food sensitivity test and determine any foods you may be allergic to and need to avoid. Wheat, dairy, yeast and sugar are often problematic and should be avoided. Substitute other grains; the sugar substitutes listed above and almond milk are all effective substitutes.
3) Focus on whole natural foods; don't eat foods that contain chemicals and preservatives.
4) Eat Omega 3 (anti-inflammatory) fats, such as wild salmon fish, Omega 3 eggs, walnuts and substitute (pro-inflammatory) meats such as beef, pork and chicken with SVP (soy vegetable protein) such as Amy's organic foods found in the grocery store – they are delicious.
5) Avoid foods containing gluten
6) Obtain protein from healthy grains and cereals, beans and legumes, healthy fish (salmon) and eggs (Omega 3). Avoid the unhealthy fats in red meat, dairy and other pro-inflammatory sources.
7) Eat lots of fresh fruit, vegetables, grains, legumes, nuts and seeds. Your liver will love you.
8) Some of the most liver-friendly foods you can eat are: carrots, celery, beets, watermelon, dark green vegetables, super foods like wheatgrass and watercress along with most vegetables , fruits, grains, nuts and legumes. Focus your meal planning on these foods and you will lose weight and be healthy. Use

only sea salt, Omega 3 fats, cook with Grapeseed oil or use the Foreman grill and avoid cooking with oil altogether and refer to the sugar substitutes above, d-ribose and Stevia for instance, are good choices, avoid processed sugar. As you can see wellness or good health, liver health and weight loss have much in common. That is how I lost 200 pounds and have kept it off for several years. Wellness is weight loss.

Achieving the Perfect pH Balance

The following food, water, supplements and therapy is recommended to achieve perfect total body pH balance (7.4) with minimal or no Herxheimer Effect.

A. Diet (emphasize the following foods)
1. Potatoes, Sweet Potatoes
2. Green Vegetables (watercress – very important)
3. Corn
4. Bananas
5. Almonds
6. Almond Milk
7. Raisins
8. Black Olives
9. Avocados
10. Flax, Olive and Coconut Oils (unheated)
11. Apricots
12. Dates
13. Brazil Nuts
14. Broccoli
15. Spinach
16. Carrots
17. Red Cabbage
18. Zucchini
19. Cucumber
20. Squash
21. Cauliflower
22. Onions
23. Garlic
24. Radishes
25. Asparagus
26. Sea Salt

27. Herbal Tea

*Eat **organic** vegetables, fruits, nuts, beans, grains and Omega-3 fats (fish, eggs)

    B. Water (Drink half-gallon to one gallon **or** 4-8 bottles daily)

        Zephyrhills Spring Water (pH – 7.7)

        Rejuvenator Water Ionizer (pH - 8.5)

    C. Supplements

        Spirulina (5 – 10 grams daily)

        Magnesium Oil (600 mg nightly – 6 sprays or more)

    D. Therapies

        FIR Sauna (detoxification, pH and cardiovascular support)

Metabolic Weight Loss Program

1. Exercise – Daily aerobic exercise for 30 minutes or more
2. Take 600 mg of Alpha-lipoic Acid (blood sugar control)
3. Rub Magnesium Oil nightly (sleep, energy)
4. Take 2 grams of Fish Oil (fat loss)
5. Take 1 tablespoon of Diatomaceous Earth daily (appetite control)
6. FIR Sauna (fat loss) for 30 minutes daily
7. Take 2000 mg of milk thistle (liver decongestion)
8. Weekly Measurements (Fat Percentage, Weight, Blood Pressure and pH)
9. Rejuvenator Alkaline Water Ionizer (pH increase) drink 96 oz daily
10. Take 10 grams of Spirulina (95% digestible protein, fat loss)

Increasing Metabolism

1. Eat (4-6) smaller meals
2. Drink 96 ounces ionized water daily (use Rejuvenator -9.0 pH)
3. Drink green tea (with d-ribose)
4. Eat ginger, peppers, onions, garlic, cinnamon, lemons, grapefruit, legumes, nuts, seeds, fish, Omega-3 eggs (without oil and salt)
5. Use FIR sauna (30-60 minutes daily)
6. Strength training (muscle burns fat)
7. Aerobic exercise (60 minutes daily)
8. Use Rejuvenator and nascent iodine (if body temperature is low)
9. Take DE (1 heaping tablespoon daily)
10. Take Spirulina (10 grams daily)

Anti-Aging

Diseases are often preventable, especially if you are eating a balanced diet consisting of only natural foods, hydrating with ionized water, using the FIR sauna to detoxify and burn fat to reach a desired fat percentage and taking the right supplements. Sadly, the Standard American Diet (SAD) is typically so far removed from wellness and anti-aging it is no wonder that so many Americans are terribly unhealthy and die prematurely. Harvard University experts and many others tell us that the human being is designed to live at least 120 years and because of recent and projected scientific discoveries, we should be able to live even longer than 120 years. Following our metabolic program combined with the hope of gene therapy and artificial organs holds the promise that one day soon we should be able to live long past 100 years (or more). It is no longer a dream, but a real possibility.

As a child, I was always amused when people would seriously consider the possibility of living to be 100 years old or beyond. What's amazing is that with the incredible work done today in the field of genetics, many problematic genes that lead to serious health problems are being identified and may be altered or eliminated. The discovery of the FOXO gene has also shown great promise for anti-aging. Many centurions have the FOXO gene in common and it may be a clue to longevity.

Our program, which includes drinking ionic water, leads to an alkaline pH and rids the body of acid waste that often causes disease and sickness. Otto Warburg, M.D. received 2 Nobel prizes for his work where he asserted that no disease can survive an alkaline pH. Combine an alkaline pH with proper body fat percentage that the FIR sauna can support, walking daily and eating only natural food, you have a wonderful combination that support anti-aging and your best protection from disease and suffering.

Strengthening Your Immune System

Your immune system consists of white blood cells, the lymphatic system or gland, adenoids, tonsils, thymus, spleen and the mucous membranes of your gastrointestinal system and respiratory tract. These organs and tissues are activated whenever you encounter microorganisms, foreign substances, allergens, pollen or animal dander. Stress, malnutrition and liver congestion can also contribute to immune dysfunction. Symptoms of a poor functioning immune system include: chronic fatigue, frequent colds, and flu or sinus infections.

To help fight infection and boost your immune system, be sure to get all the vitamins and minerals (especially vitamins A, C and E). These are important antioxidant vitamins. Eat foods such as spinach, broccoli, mango, cantaloupe, apricots, soy products, nuts and seeds and carrots to ensure you are getting the important immune boosting vitamins.

An important point to remember is that sugar is the #1 immune system depressant or enemy. Avoid sugar and consume low-glycemic fruits, d-ribose and Stevia to satisfy your "sweet tooth". Also, be sure to get 30 minutes to 2 hours daily cardiovascular exercise (including walking), get plenty of rest, use the FIR sauna 30 minutes daily, use topical magnesium nightly to help with sleep (most Americans have a magnesium deficiency) and be sure to eat natural foods and eat healthy or good fats (Omega 3, such as salmon, Omega 3 eggs, flaxseed, walnuts, etc) and avoid pro-inflammatory fats including beef, pork, dairy and poultry. Good immune boosting supplements include Colostrum, beta glucan, royal jelly and Probiotics Be sure to eat at least 30 grams of fiber daily (one serving or cup of vegetables is 4 grams, one serving of fruit is 3 grams, one serving of beans is 7 grams).

Functional Health Care

There is an amazing movement taking place in America today. National health care was just a first step and the movement towards wellness and self care continues. Health care in this country has been immersed the last 100 years trying to find the perfect medicine or machine to save lives, with some results, but little attention was ever paid to wellness and functional health care. Certainly, emergency medical personnel are much like firemen and firewomen; they save lives and are available to us 24 hours a day. That makes them valuable and important. But most Americans don't visit the fire station very often and usually do an acceptable job of fire prevention and safety on their own. We have learned what's necessary for survival, but we certainly appreciate the emergency personnel who save lives everyday and provide a valuable service to us, unfortunately little attention has been paid to what Americans badly want and need and that is prevention and wellness health care involving experts who are trained to understand both sides of health care (acute – drugs and surgery and wellness – vitamins and natural methods). The last 10 years has given birth to a new movement called "functional medicine". A new science was needed to keep America on pace with the rest of the world and help us be healthy, energetic and live longer, more productive lives. Medicine wasn't the answer alone, we needed and wanted more and the movement was essentially started with health food stores and now a health care system that is poised to recognize and encourage wellness. Functional medicine recognizes both and is "patient friendly" meaning that it does not support the 5-minute office visit and the "pill for an ill" philosophy. It supports such things as saliva testing and other functions that can be done outside the office and utilizes the Internet for communication. It is much better for the doctor and the patient. The doctor is a health care partner and advocate. It is the proverbial win-win situation and it is the best strategy available to cut costs and could even lead to balancing our budget by entirely cutting the national debt. It is a revolution that is experiencing deep resistance from pharmaceutical companies, hospitals and some insurance companies. Big money and lobbyists will continue to distort the facts, but the Internet, satellite television and cell phone technology are changing the world as we speak.

Functional medicine is certainly not new. Germany has utilized the Commission E (much like our FDA) and doctors have prescribed natural ingredients for over 50 years. We are way behind. We were the only country in the world without national health care and it is by far the best strategy to reduce or eliminate the national deficit.

Obesity and weight gain are often accompanied by guilt, frustration and much self-blame and failure thinking. It's not your fault. The commercialism of the Standard American Diet (SAD) and the absence of true wellness health care system have created the monster so many of us are facing and living with today. We need a change.

Functional health care and an understanding of nutrition, detoxification and exercise will absolutely set us free. It also is so much easier today due to products, such as water ionizers, FIR saunas, and topical magnesium oil. Functional health care will set you free, give you control and make the doctor's office visit a pleasant experience.

Maintaining your ideal weight and proper body fat percentage can be an easy experience. I've done it for over 4 years now and will keep my ideal weight the rest of my life. You can too. Functional health care is changing America. It can help change your life by visiting an Osteopath or other trained physician that specializes in functional health care. It is a movement whose time has come.

Bad Fats vs. Good Fats

Many people attempting to lose weight poor understand the role fats play in their diet. The Standard American Diet (SAD) is loaded with bad fats which cause the liver to be clogged and inefficient and inflammatory fats (meats and cheese) lead to inflammation and clogged arteries which cause obesity and diseases such as heart attacks and strokes. The liver can become severely congested and the intestines become clogged and even diseased, certainly not functional. Even "fatty liver" a phenomenon seen mostly in alcoholics is present, even rampant and causes many people to struggle with weight loss.

Cleansing your liver and eating anti-inflammatory fats (Omega 3) are extremely important as well as eating a liver-friendly diet consisting primarily of fruits, vegetables, whole grains, legumes, nuts and seeds. A liver-friendly food guide is listed in this book. Enhancing the liver's ability to process food properly will help you lose weight and improve your overall health.

If you experience poor memory, depression, joint pain, hair loss, fatigue, high cholesterol, triglycerides, hair loss, fatigue, itchy skin and poor metabolism you are probably eating too many bad fats and foods that are simply not "liver-friendly." An unfriendly liver can certainly make losing weight more difficult as well as contribute to other problems that can negatively affect your progress, such as fatigue, poor sleep and concentration among other problems.

Essentially, good fats (Omega 3) and a liver-friendly diet will keep your important liver cells strong and improve your immune system. They are also very important for weight loss and staying thin and healthy. The following is a list of the good fats to help you understand which fats to eat.

Omega 3 (anti-inflammatory fats)
1. Fish – Salmon, Mackerel, Tuna, Sardines
2. Plant Foods – Leafy greens, Walnuts, Flaxseeds, Soybeans
3. Oils – (do not heat) Cod Liver, Currant, Pumpkin, Canola

Omega 6 fats
1. Seeds (sesame, sunflower, safflower, corn, currant

2. Raw Nuts
3. Legumes – Beans, Lentils, Chickpeas
4. Oils – Primrose, Borage, Gooseberry
5. Soybeans
6. Lecithin
7. Spirulina

Omega 9 fats
1. Avocados
2. Most nuts
3. Olive Oil

Saturated (pro-inflammatory bad fats)
1. Beef
2. Pork
3. Poultry (dark meat)
4. Dairy
5. Fried Foods

Digestive Enzymes

Enzymes break down food particles, store sugar in the liver, create waste products, enable iron to link up with red blood cells, make vision and enzymes convert food to energy (very important for metabolism and weight loss. There are three basic types of digestive enzymes: protease (proteins), lipase (fats) and amylase (carbohydrates). The Standard American Diet is low in enzymes and high in bad or unhealthy foods that steal enzymes, leaving us depleted and vulnerable to disease.

Alcohol, cigarettes, drugs, medicine and unhealthy foods require or cause us to deplete enzymes. Elderly people need more enzymes. This can lead to fatigue, disease, premature aging and death.

Be careful of high protein diets. Without enzymes to properly digest them, we will experience undigested bits of protein can enter the bloodstream which may lead to diseases, such as lupus, cancer, arthritis and various allergies. Enzymes can boost energy, detoxify, slow the aging process, promote weight loss, stop inflammation, fight cancer and improve circulation. Poor enzyme consumption can lead to AIDS, allergies, viruses, arthritis, cancer, autoimmune disorders, Cohn's Disease, Multiple Sclerosis, cardiovascular diseases and obesity. Enzymes help nutrient absorption, energy, disease prevention, immune enhancement and weight loss. The human body was designed for a diet consisting of primarily plant-based foods, specifically fruits, vegetables, whole grains, nuts and seeds and legumes (beans, chickpeas, lentils. Whole, raw foods without chemicals (organic) are the only foods that will provide you with vital digestive enzymes which are extremely important for digestion and daily nutrition needs as well as being very helpful at preventing disease, weight gain, and premature aging, even death. The health implications of proper enzyme consumption are staggering, the health and longevity of almost every system in your body is dependent on the proper consumption of enzymes. Proper diet with enzymes (raw fruits, vegetables, nuts or seeds) is vital for good health.

The symptoms and disease we incur every day in this country are screaming to tell us to change our diet and lifestyle, specifically to take more digestive enzymes and eat a whole food, natural diet instead of the enzyme-less junk food we consume so much of. There are millions of cases of the following problems reported every year: heartburn, irritable bowel syndrome, gallstones, indigestion, lost work and even deaths (well over 100,000) due to digestive diseases reported every year. A staggering amount. Processed food, cooking, microwaving and heating food above 118 degrees kills enzymes. Enzymes are protein molecules responsible for thousands of physiological reactions in the body. Enzymes digest foods, repair tissue and rid our bodies of dangerous toxins. Enzymes are absolutely crucial to good health and weight loss.

Blood Sugar Disorders

What is so troubling about hypoglycemia is that millions of Americans, particularly those who are overweight and have many debilitating symptoms, don't even know they have a blood sugar disorder, such as hypoglycemia. Our typical diet is absolutely loaded with processed sugar and flour, many refined foods and many Americans drink alcohol or smoke cigarettes. We are killing ourselves with the food we eat. The average American eats over 100 pounds of sugar per year. Sugar often makes up 15% of our daily diet with sodas being the biggest culprit. Unhealthy diet drinks have only added to the problem with many experts stating that they contain neurotoxins and may be as bad or worse for us than the sugared sodas. Diabetes and hypoglycemia are two western diseases that are directly related to our sugar intake.

Hypoglycemia is a disorder you may have and it is characterized by emotional highs and lows, uncontrollable hunger, fatigue and sleep problems. Also, the adrenal glands may fail to function properly which often leads to depression, anxiety, panic attacks, low energy, poor concentration, memory problems and weight gain. Hypoglycemia tends to run in families and it is often the first step towards diabetes. You have to deal with it before it worsens and could lead to insulin dependency even dialysis.

Certainly, eliminating sugar from your diet and replacing sugar with d-ribose, Stevia and low-glycemic fruits will often satisfying your" sweet tooth", but not raise blood sugar. Sugar is the absolute enemy of the immune system and has to be addressed if you are not only going to lose weight, but stay thin for the rest of your life.

It is also important to walk at least 30 minutes daily to metabolize your food without putting as much stress on your pancreas. Certain supplements such as **Chromium Picolinate and Alpha-lipoic Acid** as well as eating small, frequent meals can be very helpful (4-6 daily meals).

The Dangers of Elevated Cortisol

Stress is the disease of the 21st century. Too little exercise, eating the wrong foods (particularly bad fats, sugar and processed foods or junk food), eating too much, too much TV, poor sleeping habits, the pressure of debt and the fast-paced modern life can be overwhelming and by middle age, for most of us, we have burned ourselves out, or more accurately, we have destroyed the body our Creator gave us and we are begin the expensive, time consuming and often times painful process of finding the answer to dealing with that catch-all term we use to describe our unhealthy lifestyles – stress. The problem is that medicine, quick and easy diet foods or gimmicks that will never produce healthy, permanent results, exercise programs we never stick with (only 10% of Americans exercise on a regular basis), divorce (more divorces today than marriages) and escape activities such as having the choice of 200 television channels, commercial-free satellite radio stations, a thousand stores that will be happy to take your money and so many other activities in the richest country in the world have left us emotionally and physically broke. By escaping and denying reality we are ignoring the emphasis we should all live our lives by: **healthy relationships, wellness and prosperity**. Do we have quality, healthy relationships with people we love and trust? Are we pursuing an alkaline lifestyle by eating pure, organic fruits, vegetables, legumes, grains and nuts or seeds? Do we drink ionized water to alkalize our bodies? Do we exercise daily, since that's what our bodies need? Are we good stewards of money, instead of careless spenders with no real priorities or goals? Life in America has gotten out of control and with your attention and effort to set your priorities and make good choices; you can control stress, be happy and relaxed and ultimately immunize yourself from stress.

The modern lifestyle may stress your adrenal glands (on top of your kidneys), produce too much cortisol (also called the "death hormone"). Unmanaged stress, junk food, especially sugar, and weight gain produce an acidic pH, which leads to oxidation, which then may lead to disease. It's not as simple as stress requiring meditation or relaxation and a few other minor changes. Let's look it at from another perspective. Otto Warburg, M.D., won the Nobel prize for proving that all disease **cannot survive** in an alkaline pH. I have had the opportunity to witness the pH levels of terminally ill patients (Cancer and AIDS) and in all cases, there pH was very low or acidic.

An elevated cortisol level is a disturbing sign that you are living a stressed life and you have to make changes quickly. A good next step is measure your pH with a test strip you can get at a health food or drug store. You will probably find numbers below 7 which indicates your body's pH is acidic and combined with an elevated cortisol level; you are living an unhealthy life that could become very problematic.

Take these steps to address the potential problems associated with stress. Be sure to take the "stress vitamins – B-Complex and C.: Use an FIR sauna to relax your body and detoxify your immune system. Drink 9.5 alkalized ionic water. Take magnesium gel or oil every night to help you sleep better and magnesium has 325 functions to help you stay healthy.. Grape Seed Extract, 300 milligrams daily, has been proven with humans to reduce blood pressure, often a problem associated with elevated cortisol. Also, walk everyday and try Yoga to stretch and relax. Listening to New Age music can also be very helpful. Avoid caffeine and anything else that may prevent relaxation. Finally, eat natural, healthy food and avoid sugar and junk food. Your body hates junk food and was not designed to metabolize it. It is poison to your body.

The Metabolic Syndrome

One of the most prevalent disorders associated with modern American life and the Standard American Diet is the Metabolic Syndrome. Our desire for fast food, artificial foods and a stressful lifestyle often lead to hypertension, blood sugar disorders and weight gain. Essentially, our metabolism becomes impaired and weight gain becomes easy. Have you ever said, "I just have to look at food and I'll gain weight." One of the real disservices we are exposed to is that many of us are led to believe that this is a normal part of aging and we typically continue our unhealthy lifestyles and take medicine or reach for anything that we think may solve the problem. Sadly, even medicine can be ineffective and blood pressure and sugar levels may never be normalized.

The key to understanding metabolic syndrome is to realize that metabolism is the key function and it has been impaired because we have essentially abused our liver and pancreas. The Standard American Diet is loaded with food that is harmful to these organs and will ultimately impair our metabolism. Preventing Metabolic Syndrome by addressing the liver and pancreas is the key. **Milk Thistle** and Dandelion are the two best herbs to detoxify and support the liver. A good dose is usually about 2000 mg daily. The liver has over 500 functions and giving it what it needs is a very good place to start. Also consider Alpha-lipoic Acid to support the pancreas. A good dose is about 600 mg daily. As always, diet plays a major part in achieving wellness. A liver friendly diet consisting of green foods, carrots, beets and other organic natural foods is your best choice. Spirulina is a great herb to get the protein you need and it is high in chlorophyll which will cleanse your liver and pancreas. I take 10 grams a day.

Drinking plenty of high quality alkaline water, daily exercise, a good detox and plenty of rest and relaxation are also helpful. If you have Metabolic Syndrome, you must eliminate unhealthy foods, such as sugar, iodized salt, bad fats, junk food and processed food. Follow the meal plan and use the recipes at 3abn.org. The Metabolic Syndrome can lead to serious problems and is not to be taken lightly. You have to make changes if you want wellness and weight loss.

The Leaky Gut Syndrome

"Leaky Gut" can be painful and lead to many other problems. I had a very bad case of the "leaky gut syndrome" a few years ago, which is basically a phenomenon in which yeast becomes prolific and seeps outside the gut and becomes blood borne. The yeast then travels to other parts of the body including the liver and digestive system. It is also responsible at times for sinus and allergic conditions. These problems are often perpetuated by sugar, yeast or alcohol in the diet. The nutrients that are often helpful include **oil of oregano, olive leaf extract and beta glucan**. Just as important, the elimination of sugar and yeast are required for at least 4 weeks until the yeast and any other toxic microorganisms are dead and no longer a threat. Taking a good Probiotics is also important to fight the toxins that have caused the gut to be out of balance. A good **Probiotics** should be at least 10 billion CFU and contain both Lactobacillus and Bifidobacteria strains (the healthy strains of bacteria) and prebiotics to feed the Probiotics, such as FOS, is also a good idea. It's always a good idea to begin a painless detoxification by taking **Diatomaceous Earth** – 1 heaping tablespoon daily (earthworkshealth.com). After about 90 days, you should experience great relief.

Leaky gut is a problem many Americans have and are unaware of. It comes primarily from poor diet, especially sugar, and can be rectified, but remember there are billions of toxic microorganisms, especially when you consume a junk food diet. You have to eat healthy food and abstain from junk food or the proliferation of yeast can spread and cause many problems, such as hardening and narrowing of the arteries, blockages, a proliferation of free radicals and immune dysfunction. The leaky gut syndrome is serious and should be addressed immediately before problems quickly occur.

Inflammation and Free Radicals

The two biggest obstacles to weight loss and wellness for most people are inflammation and free radical damage. Often times, the most significant contributor to immune dysfunction are what you eat. Due to your diet, specifically red meat, sugar, artificial foods (junk food) internal inflammation occurs which often times will lead to increased free radical activity. This will often lead to poor health, including obesity and premature aging. It is a very common occurrence in America; a very sad byproduct of an affluent society. Inflammation may produce arthritis, dermatitis, periodontal disease, cardiovascular disease and cancer. Imagine placing a drop of red dye in a glass of water. The dye will spread and eventually the entire glass of water will turn red. This is how inflammation works. It can circulate throughout the whole body and cause problems such as diabetes and cardiovascular disease. Hardening of the arteries caused by junk food and lack of exercise can cause damage to artery walls. This may trigger inflammation that may lead to heart attack or strokes. Inflammation may also complicate diabetes, even create it or make it worse.

Some of the steps you can take: Have your dentist check for and treat gum infection. Lose weight – obesity leads to inflammation. See your doctor for a checkup. Check for virus, allergy or cancer. Stop smoking – it produces inflammation and free radicals. Walking 30 minutes a day is an effective inflammation reducer. Use non-toxic cleaning products whenever possible – grapefruit seed extract is a good product to use. Eat fish and take fish oil and flaxseed oil (omega 3 anti-inflammatory fats). Avoid sugar – it is an enemy of the immune system.

Inflammation is a 21st century epidemic in this country and is the cause of cardiovascular disease, cancer and premature aging in many cases. It is important to eat anti-inflammatory fats (Omega 3), natural foods, never processed foods, quit smoking and walk when you can. The FIR sauna is an excellent tool to detox and cleanse your body of harmful toxins that my lead to inflammation and disease. FIR saunas also burn body fat, another cause of inflammation.

Grocery List

1. **Fruits** – Acai, Apples (Granny Smith – 40% less sugar), Berries, Cherries, Cantaloupes, Coconuts, Cranberries., Bananas (once a week), Citrus, Peaches, Pears, Papayas, Pomegranates Mangoes, Raisins, Watermelons, Kiwi, Pineapples (once weekly)
2. **Vegetables** – Watercress, Sweet Potatoes, Carrots, Celery, Tomatoes, Broccoli, Cauliflower, Onions, Peppers, Garlic, Cabbage, Sprouts. Chives, Cucumbers, Squash, Spinach, Beets, Olives, Zucchini, Eggplant, Lettuce
3. **Fish** – Wild Salmon, Tuna (small), Ocean Fish (small)
4. **Soy** – Edamame, SVP, Tofu, Tempeh, Milk and Cheese
5. **Beverages** – Almond Milk, Green Tea, Organic Decaf Coffee (2 cups), 100% Juice
6. **Grains** - Quinoa, Oatmeal, Brown Rice, Whole Grains, Bread- Alvarado St., Ezekiel
7. **Cereals** - Nature's Path, Arrowhead Mills, Ezekiel, Kashi
8. **Spices** – Cinnamon, Curry, Pepper, Sea Salt
9. **Oils** – Flaxseed, Olive Oil, Coconut Oil, Grapeseed, Macadamia
10. **Legumes** – Beans, Chickpeas, Sweet and Split Peas, Lentils, **Hummus Pine Nut,** Garlic

11. **Nuts** – (No oil or salt) Walnuts, Pecans, Almonds, Flaxseeds Sunflower Seeds
12. **Protein** – Omega 3 Eggs, Fish, Legumes, Grains
13. **Sweeteners** – D-Ribose, Stevia, Buckwheat Honey, Maple Syrup
14. **Frozen Foods** – **Amy's**, Kashi's
15. **Yogurt** – Stonyfield
16. **Meats** – Fish (salmon, tuna), Chicken and Turkey Breast

Meal Plan

Breakfast

Oatmeal or Quinoa (with d-ribose, Stevia, buckwheat honey or maple syrup)
Dried Cranberries, Raisins, Walnuts   (or)
Brown rice with Omega-3 eggs (2)   (or)
Cereal (see list for approved cereals)
(Plus)   Fruit (mango, berries, or orange)

Lunch
Soup – sea salt, 6 or more vegetables   (or)
Tuna or Egg Salad (use approved mayonnaise) with vegetables (use approved bread)
(Plus) Fruit – Apple or berries

Dinner
Salmon with Quinoa or Brown Rice
Salad – 6 vegetables or more (with approved salad dressing)
Mango or berries

Snack
Carrots, Celery, Brown Rice Cakes, and Chocolate Candy Bar (see Wellness Bakery)

Beverages
Green Tea, Organic Decaffeinated Coffee (2 cups limit), Acai Juice, Goji, Pomegranate, Mangosteen Juice, Pure Vegetable or Low Glycemic 100% fruit juice, Water

Sweeteners
D-ribose, Stevia, Maple Syrup, Buckwheat Honey

Recipes

When cooking, always remember to eat only natural food and make sure the big 3 are addressed properly. Never eat processed **sugar**, use Stevia, D-Ribose, fruits, buckwheat honey or molasses syrup instead. Never use iodized **salt,** such as Morton's, always use sea salt and never use oil to cook with that will convert from unsaturated to saturated fat, instead use **Grapeseed oil,** which has a high smoke point and will not convert to unhealthy saturated fat. Also, use a foreman grill to avoid cooking with oil when possible.

Go to **3abn.org** or **bioinnovations.net** to download healthy recipes.

20 Reasons to Follow This Program

1. Consistent, Easy Weight Loss – 3 pounds per week average
2. Fat Burning - Goal is 20% Total Body Fat Percentage
3. Sugar Control (Members of the American Diabetic Association)
4. Appetite Control
5. Energy Increase
6. Healthy Body Fats (omega 3)
7. Hormonal Balance
8. Cardiovascular Support (Inflammation Control)
9. Cholesterol Reduction
10. Triglycerides (Blood Fats Reduction)
11. Digestive Enzyme Increase
12. Antioxidant Increase
13. Immune Function Improvement
14. Liver Decongestion
15. Improved Digestion
16. Lowered Free Radicals
17. Improved Intestinal Function
18. Improved pH (alkalinity)
19. Hydration Improvement
20. Overall Disease Prevention

Top Twenty Tests

1. Body Fat Percentage – (Goal – 20% women, 15% men)
2. Blood Pressure – (115/75)
3. Total Cholesterol – (150-200)
4. LDL Cholesterol – (100 or less)
5. HDL Cholesterol – (60 or above)
6. LPA – 30
7. Triglycerides (100 or less)
8. Vitamin D – (100 or above Hydroxy 25)
9. SED – (30 or below)
10. C-Reactive Protein – (1 or 2)
11. AIC Hemoglobin – (6.0 or below)
12. Blood Sugar (80-100)
13. Homocysteine – (10 or below)
14. pH – 7.4 saliva
15. DMSA (heavy Metals) – 50 – 1000 mg DMSA
16. Cortisol (stress) – high after waking and low at bedtime
17. BNP (heart) – (100 or less)
18. Bowel Movements – (1-3 daily, light brown, toothpaste texture)
19. Thyroid – (97 degree body temperature or above at 6 am)
20. Fiber – 40 grams a day (Most Americans eat 10 grams)

Fat Burning Cocktail

1. Carrots   4 ounces
2. Beets   4 ounces
3. Celery   4 ounces
4. Granny Smith Apples   4 ounces
5. Watermelon   4 ounces
6. Acai (optional)   4 ounces

24 ounces daily, 168 ounces weekly

1. Juice 1 time every 2 weeks. Freeze one bottle and use the other
2. Add D-Ribose or Stevia for sweetening
3. Drink 12 ounces (twice) daily
4. Use organic fruits and vegetables when possible

This cocktail will cleanse and enhance your liver, improve immune function and increase fat burning

<u>Dining Out Guide</u>

1. **Subway**
   > 9 grain whole wheat bread
   > Tuna salad
   > All Vegetables
   > Water
   > Bring fruit for dessert

2. **Wendy's**
   > Baked Potato with Broccoli
   > Salad
   > Water
   > Bring fruit for dessert

3. **Burger King**
   > Vegetarian Burger
   > All Vegetables
   > Water
   > Bring fruit for dessert

4. **McDonald's**
   > Oatmeal
   > (or) Salad
   > Water
   > Bring fruit for dessert

5. **Chipotle's**
   > Burrito Bowl (Beans, Rice, Grilled Chicken)
   > Water
   > Bring Fruit for dessert

6. **Restaurants (Thai, Japanese, Latin)**

No fried foods
Vegetables, Fruits
Fish
Soy Foods (Edamame, tofu, miso)
Brown Rice or Quinoa (bring)
Beans, Salsa
Tea

The Wellness Bakery

1. Sweeteners - D-Ribose, Stevia, Lo Han, Buckwheat Honey, Maple Syrup
2. Oil – Grapeseed or Macadamia Nut
3. Salt – Sea Salt
4. Honey – Buckwheat
5. Whole Wheat Flour
6. Almond or Soy Milk
7. Cinnamon
8. Thickener – Arrowroot, Lecithin
9. Antioxidants – Berries, Acai, Dark Chocolate
10. Nuts and Seeds -Walnuts, Flaxseed, Pecans, Almonds, Sunflower

Products – Cookies, Cakes, Pies, Éclairs, Candies

Chocolate Candy Bars

1. Unsweetened, unprocessed non-alkalized 70% Cocoa Powder (dark chocolate)
2. Acai Juice
3. Blueberries
4. Walnuts and Almonds
5. D-Ribose (sweetener)
6. Lecithin (thickener)

The Wellness Shield

1. Acai Juice – (ORAC – 1026)
2. Green Tea – (200 times more powerful than Vitamin E, increases immune function by 500%)
3. Watercress- Repairs DNA, Scored 1000 (perfect Score) on Nutrition Test
4. Broccoli, Cabbage, Cauliflower – Indole - 3 Carbinol
5. Carrots, Tomatoes – Carotenoids
6. Onions, Apples – Quercetin
7. Soy (Edamame, Miso, Tofu) – Genistein
8. Curry- Curcumin
9. D – Ribose – Increases energy by 45%, lowers blood sugar
10. Sea Salt – 25% less sodium
11. Grapeseed, Macadamia Oils – High Smoke Point (good for cooking)
12. Flaxseed, Coconut, Olive Oils – Healthy at room temperature

- Omega-3 (anti-inflammatory fat) – Salmon, Flaxseed, Walnut, Omega-3 eggs

Appetite Suppressing Scents
4. Banana
5. Peppermint
6. Green Apple

smellandtaste.org – Allan Hirsch, M.D.

The FIR Sauna Benefits

7. **Average weight loss** – 1 pound per week (daily 30 minute sessions)
8. **Calories expended** – 600 to 2400 calories per 30 minute session
9. **Cleansing/Detoxification** – Lymphatic and Immune System
10. **Cardiovascular Benefits** – 6 mile run per 30 minute session
11. **Improves relaxation and sleep**
12. **Facial Cleansing** (reduces toxins)

The FIR Sauna is light, portable, unzips and can be washed and hung to dry, easily transported in the trunk of a small car, arm vents allows freedom to use laptop computer, phone, watch TV or listen to music.

Your sauna has been endorsed by NASA (used by the astronauts), American Heart Association, used by many hospitals, health clubs all over the world and is especially effective at **burning fat.**

Using EFT for Weight Loss-Why does it often work where nothing else will?

EFT provides several remarkable benefits for weight loss that sets it apart from other counseling methods:

Benefit #1 - EFT Can Reduce or Eliminate Your Immediate Cravings: Using EFT for 1 or 2 minutes can arrest your cravings in many cases. Thus, you may no longer need to "eat when you are not hungry." This feature surprises most newcomers. In research studies it has been found to reduce cravings quickly and reliably.

Benefit #2 - EFT Can Reduce or Eliminate Emotional Overeating: If you have been using food to "tranquilize" years of past emotional hurts, you may find EFT to be your best friend. EFT can bring you more emotional peace which, in turn, can lead to more sensible eating habits. This emotional contributor to overeating, which EFT is designed to address, is the **missing piece** in most weight loss programs.

EFT has been evaluated in several scientific studies of food cravings and weight loss, and has been found to help people with emotional overeating and cravings. In one study (published in the peer-reviewed journal *Integrative Medicine)*, EFT reduced cravings by 83%.There is a new program called Ideal Weight EFT, which uses state-of-the art scientific knowledge, powerful motivational techniques, and a supportive community. EFT is easy to apply and **can work where nothing else does.**

Additional EFT Benefits

- EFT diminishes Binge Eating in 12 sessions (on average)
- EFT eliminates major emotional barriers
- Successful weight loss can be achieved over the Phone
- Compulsive Overeating and Weight Loss Protocol
- Addresses Addiction and the Cause of Weight Loss

It's Not What You're Eating, But What's Eating You!

Living in a complicated world where competition, survival, recreation, contribution, self-esteem and security require extreme participation, but support is necessary to stay competitive and remain relevant. It is very hard to know what support you need to stay competitive and where it will come from. It is easy to feel all alone and completely unsupported in this diverse and very competitive society. We can't enjoy, much less sustain, success without adequate support. We will quickly become frustrated, lonely, confused and feel virtually irrelevant. Support must come from three sources: 1) Your Creator   2) Your Significant Others (family, etc.)   3) Your Employment. Your Creator can provide you with leadership, strength, and a blueprint or a guidepost and example to lead and mold your life. Some people believe prayer is a good way to communicate or clarify your desires and plans. Your Creator helps you and can be the best partner and understanding friend you will ever have. Your family must be an absolute priority in a changing, potentially hostile and competitive world. Without them, we become ineffective and often weak and feel unimportant. They are never perfect, but they should receive our unconditional love or else you will never know the joy and peace of family, or significant others. Don't expect perfection because they can't give it to you. The comfort and peace of a supportive family is an absolute necessity in a stressful, competitive world. Work is a means to fulfill expression. Work is a need to support others, security, a feeling of being needed, useful and relevant. Without work we find our role and function in society to be questionable. We question our value and purpose in life. We must express and participate and fill a need no one else can provide for us.

Life requires support.

Weight Loss Builds Self Esteem

Most of our disappointments and failures in life come as a result of low self confidence. Weight gain is no exception. Almost every important thing to us requires self confidence such as success in school, jobs, marriages and parenting. Yes, losing weight and staying thin permanently takes self confidence and perseverance. As an adult you have to walk and chew gum so to speak at the same time. Whether we like it or not we have to earn money, have some relationships and many of us support marriages and families. We have to maintain some competency in all of these areas plus stay healthy otherwise poor health and stress can be absolutely overwhelming. We must take the time to honestly review and consider our family, school, friendships, work and romances. Often times, we would rather forget unpleasant experiences. We may not even remember that much about our childhood. Chances are though that you probably still have a few skeletons in the closet. I certainly did. If only we would look like skeletons instead of feel like skeletons. My self confidence journey began when I was in the 5th grade. For four years I had to deal with unruly kids who wanted to fight everyday. Not to mention I had little interest in school or belief in myself. My weight started to escalate in the 3rd grade and I was labeled as a "fat kid". I eventually became the smart, fat kid who never really got over these early painful years. I just stuffed the painful memories and believed I was "less than" everyone else and I would never realize the benefits thin people would enjoy. Like most kids, I really wanted to be thin and popular, especially with the girls. Being a fat kid is a tough life. As an adult, I wished many times I could go back to those early years and become the most popular kid in school.

Childhood disappointments, parental conflicts and unresolved situations are the breeding ground for adult habits and addictions, like obesity that often lead to lifelong habits as an adult that are typically misunderstood and unresolved. Being thin and well is for everyone and it is possible for you. The solution is clear. Achieving everything you want and anything of value you must understand the problem and develop the self confidence and perseverance to know you can be successful. Not just for a select few, but for everyone – I'm living proof. Wellness is the answer.

To gain self confidence, realize you were not made to fail, but made by a Creator who deeply loves you and created a friendly universe for us all. Remember, "I prosper everyone and everyone prospers me." Much like Dorothy in the movie "The Wizard of Oz" you could always go home or "back to Kansas" you simply lacked the self confidence and belief that it was truly possible. As you will learn throughout this book, let go, image your success, affirm it often and then use the perseverance which has gotten you through so many things in life. Don't accept failure, never give up and be passionate about wellness. Radiate success and you will attract it.

Love is Appreciation

If you really love someone, you deeply appreciate them for all they do for you. Love is caring, understanding, and recognizing our unique lifestyles and what we need; what makes us work or operate. It is not easy for us to be appreciated, but to truly love us means cutting through the façade we often employ to be noticed, accepted and ultimately appreciated.

We don't have to be bribed, induced or persuaded by anyone to genuinely be loved. We know we are fully appreciated and respected for who we are. It has nothing to do with how we look, how much we are worth or what we can provide. We can truly love someone for simply being their self. We should always appreciate the people we love. Feeling unappreciated and exploited often leads to low self-esteem and depression. This situation is typically a breeding ground for obesity and illness. You have to begin appreciating others and demonstrate the value and worth of appreciation and ultimately respect. If you're still not receiving appreciation, you have to demand it. Everyone deserves respect and appreciation. It is vital to good health. You should never stay in a hopeless situation where you feel you'll never be respected no matter what you do.

Contentment

For many of us, weight gain or poor weight management is a result of being dissatisfied, unhappy and lacking self control. What do we really want or need? Our unfulfilled lives and lack of clear understanding about what we really want or need and what makes us truly happy leaves us pursuing temporary pleasure, following the status quo, feeling trapped in conventional wisdom and longing for guidance, peace, and prosperity. We want to discover joy, purpose, love, satisfaction and contentment. We want to lead a fulfilling life that reflects our values, desires, needs and beliefs. We also want to make a difference, help people and leave the world with a favorable, lasting impression of us. This all may sound like an impossible dream, but we only have one life to live and I think it is important to discover ourselves, take chances, make sacrifices and be very clear about who we really are and want and what it takes for us to lead a satisfying, prosperous and content life,

Many questions must be answered before we can find our own space in the world. The following questions are a good starting point.

1. What is your relationship with the Creator?
2. Are you a giver and helper? Are you a giver and helper?
3. What more can you be?
4. Are you a good role model?
5. What do you lack or need?

6. What is important to you and what do really care about?
7. What do you need?
8. Are you willing to sacrifice to grow?
9. What's been holding you back?
10. Do you accept and love yourself?

Self acceptance is difficult, because the world will always tell you to be better and there is so much more for you to do. This notion is primarily driven by the advertising community and its sole purpose is financial. In other words, this is the essence of marketing in America. Ignore it. Focus on you and achieving prosperity, which is an internal function. Once you finally accept and love yourself, you will have achieved the highest possible function you can achieve. It doesn't matter what others say, because they are just as lost or want something, such as your money. Love, acceptance and true contentment are personal and only you can have it for yourself. You are loved and accepted by your Creator and the Universe is a friendly and loving place. Contentment is achieved through the mind. There are only three functions on earth: relationships (God, family, friends), wellness and prosperity. Your mind should be cleared and focused on making these three areas acceptable to you and then set out to do what you believe you need to do in order to satisfy your time here. It isn't hard; it's just unusual because most people never reach this point in their lives. Love yourself. Accept yourself and remember you are actually surrounded by love in this Universe. Choose to accept it.

Birth Order

We can't choose our birth order, but did you know there are strong characteristics and tendencies linked to the order in which you were born?
First born children are often strong-willed, compulsive, high achieving leaders and will often suffer from stress-related problems, such as alcoholism, food addiction and cardiovascular disease. It is an interesting fact that over 95% of American presidents and Fortune 500 Company CEO's are first born children. Divorce rates are very high and mixed with the privileges many first-born children enjoy are many adult problems occur.

Middle children are often less decisive and procrastinators. They are not typically leaders, compared to first born children, but often prefer sure choices, stability and security. Typically, they are less mobile and not as progressive. They often don't have the attention and pressure the first born child experienced, but having less pressure also may lead to a more relaxed adulthood and more acceptance with less stress.

Babies and only children are usually the best adjusted and may have the most satisfying lives. They have less pressure growing up and, much like the first born; they receive the attention and feel the acceptance without the stress of performance and achievement. They tend to be more accepting and are often the best adjusted child that leads a satisfying life. Competition and failure avoidance, key to many first born children, are not nearly as important and relevant issues to babies.

Often times, our birth order will dictate our choices and consequences in adulthood. Older, first born children, for instance may experience a higher incidence of alcoholism and divorce. The shoulds and musts we lived with as children may invoke or cultivate habits or choices that become problematic. If we were told that successful people should go to college, successfully marry, earn a certain income or look certain way, but we never live up to those expectations, we believe we are a failure or we lack what is necessary to be happy and successful. Obesity can be particularly painful and discomforting. Stinking thinking (depression and anxiety we often feel) is perpetuated by the "shoulds and musts" generated from childhood. It's important to recognize the "stinking thinking" and not let your decisions and life choice much better to choose rational, healthy and constructive choices that lead to productive results
If you are like many people, obesity is something you blame on an inability to control appetite, poor self esteem and lack of control generally. It's your fault and anytime you want to you will control your appetite, be thin and healthy. For the last 50 years, AA and other groups have used support, group therapy and a disease model as the foundation of its

treatment program, but have failed to realize the significance of the body's natural chemical makeup and its importance. There are two basic neurotransmitters that control our emotional state: serotonin for depression and dopamine for anxiety. A disruption with either can lead to anxiety, depression, addictive behaviors and other problems. The gut controls 90% of our moods and combined with toxicity (bad foods, etc) can be a major contributor to our moods and health. The following is an appropriate and effective plan for weight loss and wellness that addresses the underlying junk food addiction.

5-HTP   (neurotransmitter support for depression)
Probiotics   (supports gut health)
FIR Sauna   (detoxification and immune support)
Magnesium crème or oil   (relaxation)

The above elements have rarely, if ever, been used for addictive behavior control. Sadly, junk food addiction is not considered an addiction by the medical community. Our birth order can be a prerequisite or contributing factor to adult addiction and many times, the wellness approach of diet, nutrition, detoxification and prosperity thinking along with the psychological explanation of past events that led to current functioning is the answer that so many people need. They need to understand that it's not their fault and the current addictive behavior is explainable and can be addressed.

Males vs. Females

Some things cannot be changed. Our birth sex yields often predictable characteristics that can be easily managed with proper knowledge and a good plan or can become problematic and yield problems, sometimes for life. Many people will experience characteristics from an early age indicative of sexual orientation and not necessarily of personality. Young girls may be oriented towards "Ken and Barbie", perfect or ideal families, animals, etc that typify harmony or positive interaction. Males often may prefer sports or some interaction that requires competition and physical activity. Hedonism or pleasure seeking may be a motivating force that will ultimately set the tone for adult behavior. It is easy to see the potential conflicts between the sexes that may lead to future discord.

As the sexes mature, sexual behavior can be conflicting and confusing. Based on characteristics that formed personality styles (as described above), women often prefer longer, more involved pre-sexual interaction than men. That is why women are sometimes described as "crockpots" and men may closely resemble "microwave ovens" in terms of how they approach sexual relations. One day, the microwave oven will marry the crockpot though and different cooking temperatures may result in visits to the marriage counselor's office. Successful relationships are **made** and not typically **found**. Significant others are a special gift, just as our children are. Often

times, money and assertive communication are given as the cause of the problem.
We must understand we are different and we should compliment each other and not conflict with each other. Love is a great gift and it's worth the effort to "change the oil" and get a new perspective and learn to accept and conquer our differences.

The 4 M's and the 1 M

We are taught from an early age that "if it is to be it is up to me'. The 10 magic 2 letter words. Trusting anyone can be a very difficult and even frightening experience that many of us avoid. We're taught it is simply better to do it ourselves, because most people will ultimately let us down. But then life becomes so complicated and difficult and we need a savior to help us deal with our problems and plan our future. Trust and disappointment are the most difficult issues most people struggle with.
By accepting the 4 m's, most of us have been raised to believe (man – message – monument – machine) we fail realize this we an invention of the early church and still exists today. In the case of Christianity, this can be explained as Jesus – bible – cross – church). It was used to keep the masses or people at bay so the privileged few at the top would maintain control. It is simply not the truth and the truth that we must embrace is that love fulfills the whole law, our Creator is simply love and love is our Creator.

The 1 M is about the **message** and that
message is **love**. Certainly, the bible says this
and Paul in Corinthians stated that in the end
there is only hope, faith and love and love is the
greatest of all. Believing in the 4 m's can be
destructive and very limiting, not to mention
not true. Set your course on radiating love and
you will attract it in its many forms. It is the
only M that will liberate you can help you find
true prosperity.

Humility

It is common during childhood to defend our
ego, assert ourselves or to crave, even demand
attention and respect. As we become teenagers
and young adults, our challenge is often to "fit
in" or find ourselves and stake out a place or
position for our unique selves. As we grow
older, we are often faced with "identity crisis."
We try to fit in, experience dissatisfaction with
jobs, marriages and even life. We also make
mistakes because we do not fully understand
ourselves or worse we have a hard time just
being ourselves and loving ourselves.. What's
the solution? How do we live a rich, satisfying
happy and peaceful life? We must follow these
steps:

1. Love your Creator and understand who
   He made (you) to be. Be thankful and
   always seek His advice on important
   matters.
2. Give. Learn to be a giver. Be a giver
   instead of a selfish taker. Think of the
   people you love and the people you can

help by giving. You are always supported by your Heavenly Father which allows you to freely give.

3. Help others, especially significant others, such as your family members. Help them to feel good about themselves. Give them compliments. Tell them positive things about themselves instead of focusing on the negative events in life as most of us do. The world is a negative, challenging place. We all have a desperate need for someone (like you) to help us through the rough spots.

4. Be humble. Give your time and talent to people whenever possible. Lift people up. It will help you feel loved, needed and connected.

If you are a parent, follow these tips for a stronger relationship:

1. Teach your children what you feel is important and necessary. No one else can do it better than you.

2. Be proactive – organize and plan your days. Remember, there are only a few areas (money, relationships, school, spiritual, health) that you should be primarily concerned with. Always choose quality over quantity.

3. Be consistent. As a therapist, I felt inconsistency was the main problem I saw that lead to misunderstandings and problematic behavior.

4. Focus and prioritize. Mothers especially have trouble with this one because they are overextended and absolutely must be assertive to achieve optimum focus. You may also need help – you can't do it all!
5. Network with helpful, successful people you trust
6. Get organized – write everything down, use your computer and remember to prioritize daily every event
7. Reduce or eliminate difficult problems such as debt, an unreliable car and household appliances, unproductive friends and acquaintances and any bad habits. You don't have time for unnecessary people and functions in your life. Follow the Personal Finance First Aid Kit to improve your financial situation.
8. Limit your child's television time and choose programs carefully.
9. Create balance for your children. Try many different sports, spiritual activities, reading good books and "play" with your children. They love to spend time with their parents.
10. If broken and if possible, work on your marriage Children are special and a real blessing, but they also require time and money and can be a real strain on marriages if you are unprepared or unable to deal with the stress and pressure. Whatever

you can do to help your marriage, a night for each other, a short vacation or trip, an extra job (if needed) or time together in church or fun activities, but a healthy marriage is critical for parenting, when possible.

11. Meditate when possible and use affirmations daily. They can be very effective.
12. Don't try to live up to your parents or any other role model. Be yourself!
13. As a parent, you are a role model. Always be aware of your activities and conduct around your children.
14. Being a parent is the greatest job in the world! Be thankful every day.

Frustration Tolerance

Frustration tolerance defines us. We all hate to be frustrated. We all usually avoid it an d there are many alternatives to frustration such as unhealthy food, movies, TV, music and simply playing or unfortunately illegal behavior and unhealthy activities to fill the void and help us avoid frustration. We may "self-medicate" with drugs or alcohol or abandon relationships, jobs or other responsibilities because we simply can't tolerate frustration. The older we get the more we despise and avoid frustration. It can even kill us when we become helpless, overwhelmed and "fed up" with our complicated unsatisfying and depressing lives. Self-medication becomes overeating junk food and escape activities such as oversleeping, sexual affairs and careless spending. Fantasy and "feel good" are the activities of choice and patience, achievement and wise choices are often not chosen. It becomes a hopeless and vicious circle. .I've been frustrated and I hated it. I felt so out of control.

Frustration is about choices. It is about commitment. It is a pass-fail experience with no safe, easy middle-of-the-road choices. It is a win or lose situation. My choices that saved my life was to see life in a spiritual and uplifting way. I chose love, family, wellness (by eating healthy, natural food), giving, caring, sharing and helping others. Our Creator's plan for us is joy (better than happiness), eternal life and a satisfying life greater than I could have ever imagined. We can give all of our problems to a higher being who is absolutely the best friend you will ever have. You can't go wrong. Frustration is difficult to manage, much less tolerate. You need a mentor, a friend and an advisor.

Weight reduction and management can be very frustrating. That's why you have to simplify and focus on your objectives. For me, I focused on healing important relationships (family), dissolving a few unnecessary relationships, wellness (eating natural food, walking, drinking enough water, sleeping well, taking the right supplements and prosperity (financial peace and good stewardship). Follow this program and you will get there. However long it takes, you're moving in the right direction. Don't put pressure on yourself (as most dieters do) and think of yourself as the long distance runner who will finish the race, instead of the sprinter who looks good and starts out well, but will never finish the weight loss race and will chalk up the loss to another faulty program. This is your program and your life. Don't stop until you cross the finish line. I did and so can you.

Activating Your Desires

Most of us never obtain our desires and many people aren't even sure exactly what they desire. Use the following guidelines to understand your desires and go after them. You will be amazed how much your life can change.

1. Go from "I can't" to "Yes I can"
2. The resistance behind (no I can't" largely comes from the world and dead past or unborn future issues. Make today the only day that matters.
3. Use imaging, prayer, affirmations to help you get past failure and dead past issues.

4. Look at your health in an entirely different way. Think of critical care medical personnel (doctors, etc) as firemen and women who help us when we need the help, but let's face it, how often do you go to the fire station when your house is safe and not on fire? Not very often I'm sure. Seek out functional doctors (such as Osteopaths and others that understand wellness health care), learn about health care by studying this book and be your own doctor. Commit to leading a wellness lifestyle so you are thin, fit and healthy. You'll love it.

5. Be a good steward. Manage your debt (avoid debt when possible) and increase your rating score (FICO) so you'll feel better and can obtain money if you need it.

6. Be proactive instead of reactive. Have a prosperity plan, go after what you really want, image, pray and affirm it. No more blame, failure, pessimism. It can be done and it will be done. Don't accept failure under any circumstances.

7. Learn to be assertive. Say what you mean and mean what you say. Get the right timing, tone of voice and a constructive message to ensure assertiveness. You are like a pitcher in a baseball game. You have to use many good pitches and there will be many effective batters you face. It is also a long game and you will be hit and lose games. No pitcher is perfect. The key is discipline, patience and confidence. It

isn't easy, but it's important and you will always be much happier when you learn to be assertive.

8. Love is to be made and not found. What seemed so important in our 20's will quickly fade. We all wish our spouse were our best friends. Assertive communication, patience, addressing key issues such as children, finances and living situations are always necessary. This is the "making" of love and it takes time and patience. You have to be unselfish realizing that the payoff is a happy family, meaning children, spouse and generally helping each other through the hard times. It's worth the effort.

Emotional Modulation

In the wellness arena, autoimmune diseases such as Multiple Sclerosis and Lupus are diseases in which the body is actually attacking itself. Your body is overreacting or overprotecting itself which may lead to negative results. Your immune system can be weakened by many diseases, including autoimmune diseases, and is unable to fight them off and defend itself against such attacks or problems.

Thinking right thoughts is emotional modulation. Avoiding "stinking thinking" is an example of positive emotional modulation. Affirmations, imaging and making right choices leads to healthy emotional modulation. Right or healthy living and making rational, healthy decisions lead to a balanced lifestyle. It takes discipline, patience and commitment. Emotional modulation and living a life filled with peace and joy and is a choice and a decision. You must renew your mind and dissolve previous issues that are still hanging around and greatly influencing your decisions, even when you don't realize it. They can be automatic and very stubborn. Parental influence can be a place to start as you identify the issues and influences that are preventing you from being objective and constructive.

Modulation is an experience that commits you to living a life filled with peace and joy. It is a choice and will ultimately help you find balance and truth in your life. It is an immersion or total experience to be absolutely involved or committed to peace, joy and love. Depression, anxiety, doubt, fear and other problematic emotions often result from a lack of focus, commitment and appreciation of healthy choices. Life requires discipline, trust and belief to succeed.

We must "crowd" out" the negative, destructive thoughts with pure, uplifting thoughts. Much like our lawns, we need emotional "fertilizer" to build the grass (or positive thoughts) and "weed killer" (avoidance) to dissolve the negative and destructive thought processes we have all experienced and disliked. Your joy begins with your cognitive or thought processes. You have to get it right in the mind first. Your actions will follow. Flood yourself with thoughts and actions of giving, praying, imaging and affirmations.

The final step is passionate persistence. Never give up. Once you have committed and abide in what you know is right, your persistence will modulate or balance your emotions and ultimately help you achieve your goals.

Assertive Communication

Probably one of the most cited reasons for relationship failure is passive-aggressive or nonassertive communication. Parenting, marriage and work-related relationships depend on it. Most of us surrender too soon and too easily to confrontation and discord. Anger, stress, financial pressure and physical impairment are very likely to produce poor communication which may lead to disastrous results and we don't know how to resolve it. It becomes very hard to escape and maintain a relationship. It becomes an endless challenge with poor results.

Remember, there are a few elements that will help you and when used correctly will greatly improve your life.

1, Always use proper timing. Now is almost always the best time. Do not wait unless it is important to take a time out to calm down and be constructive. Don't be passive and let unresolved issues linger and build. This is how passive-aggressive communication occurs.

2. Use a proper and constructive tone of voice. Not too passive. Talk plainly, clearly, be fair, honest, do not yell or scream. Be assertive – in the middle, calm down and be constructive.

You always want a good result and to be able to finish on a positive note. I know this can be hard, but by insisting on healthy, assertive communication all the time, you create a very positive and constructive habit or pattern that shapes your relationship and becomes natural, but it can take awhile. It's worth the effort.

3. The proper message is always important. Be constructive, clear, fair and honest. You have to be trusted and credible. Many couples let their emotions rule and they often fight with no constructive message which may produce very complicated conditions.

4. Ask questions. Psychologists receive a lot of money to ask good, meaningful questions. Pull the other person in and let them tell you what they want to say. A dialogue may produce other pertinent and relative questions or points to be made. Don't be afraid to be assertive. I really believe the truth will set you free. If your partner can't be truthful or doesn't want to know the truth, there is no relationship. Never be afraid to be assertive, especially with family members. Most problems can usually be solved with assertive communication, but it takes patients and a commitment to honesty with a desire for constructive communication. It's not easy, but worth it.

Controlling Food Addiction

We live in denial and slowly waste our lives by eating unhealthy food, not drinking enough water, not getting the proper nutrition we need and most of us (90% nationally) never exercise regularly. Because we simply don't realize how bad things can get and how quickly they can deteriorate, we minimize or basically ignore the reality of what we must do to be healthy, happy and well.

We simply can't allow ourselves to binge on sugar, unhealthy fat (pro-inflammatory) and eat foods that slowly destroy our bodies. We become much like alcoholics and drug addicts – we keep destroying our bodies. We give ourselves permission to self-destruct because it the easiest and most desirable (at the time) choice because we are basically hedonistic – we seek pleasure, not discipline. We satisfy our heads (mouth for taste, nose for smell, eyes for sight) and not our body organs which want nutritious foods, not junk food. We keep destroying our bodies, until it's too late. We often ignore the reality that everything we value in our lives required us to exercise discipline – school diplomas, children, marriage, a meaningful promotion at work, a home (paying off a 30-year mortgage). They all took time and discipline. The best things in life take a great deal of effort and patience. They are not easy, quick or simple, but we appreciate them.

As they say easy come and easy go. You must make just 1 decision today and stick to it. Either choose to be well or take a chance with your health. Stop minimizing, letting yourself off the hook, rationalizing your irrational behavior and choose wellness.

Obesity is 1 of 4 major additions in this country and it's the biggest. Let this program help you balance blood sugar, experience an alkaline pH and explore the tasty, delicious and healthy foods you can eat that will change your life. I did and I wish I had made the change earlier in my life. Psychologists estimate that psychological change to break habits takes about 30 days. That is why drug and alcohol treatment centers are 30 days. You can overcome both physical and psychological addiction in 30 days. All you have to do is want it bad enough.

I have treated many alcoholics and drug addicts during the years and I know how difficult and trying treatment and abstention can be. Food addiction and weight loss and wellness can also be difficult and like drug and alcohol treatment, recidivism and failure can be very high. Over 90% of Americans who are addicted to junk food and lose weight will gain back every pound they lost and will never know the happiness of being at ideal weight for any length of time.

Treatment centers for addictions are typically 30 day programs because experts agree that it requires about 30 days to conquer any addiction from a psychological standpoint. I believe food addiction is no different. Even with ionized water, FIR saunas, great supplements and a completely natural food diet emphasizing the omega 3 fats, it will still take time to identify and manage the psychological issues that have held you back. Typically, marriages or interpersonal relationships, failed employment situations and guilt couple with poor health are usually the culprits. Begin doing what you can, such as drinking ionized water, using an FIR sauna and walking whenever you can. Take supplements for appetite control and blood sugar balance and eat a whole food, organic diet. Try to identify the issue or issues that have precipitated your obesity and be patient. It will take time and patience.

Understand that weight loss is much like flying an airplane, there's a lot to getting started and getting the plane in the air, but once you are able to level off you can assume cruising speed, so to speak, where everything becomes habit and routine. The great thing about our program is that there is no maintenance or adjustments to be made when you have reached ideal weight. You will realize that your previous acidic pH, high body fat percentage (reduced with the help of the FIR sauna), need for proper supplementation and focusing on an Omega 3 organic natural food diet will give you the blueprint you need to remain thin and well. I have treated many alcoholics and drug addicts during the years and I know how difficult and trying treatment and abstention can be.

Food addiction and weight loss and wellness can also be difficult and like drug and alcohol treatment, recidivism and failure can be very high. Over 90% of Americans who are addicted to junk food and lose weight will gain back every pound they lost and will never know the happiness of being at ideal weight for any length of time.

Treatment centers for addictions are typically 30 day programs because experts agree that it requires about 30 days to conquer any addiction from a psychological standpoint. I believe food addiction is no different. Even with ionized water, FIR saunas, great supplements and a completely natural food diet emphasizing the omega 3 fats, it will still take time to identify and manage the psychological issues that have held you back. Typically, marriages or interpersonal relationships, failed employment situations and guilt couple with poor health are usually the culprits. Begin doing what you can, such as drinking ionized water, using an FIR sauna and walking whenever you can. Take supplements for appetite control and blood sugar balance and eat a whole food, organic diet. Try to identify the issue or issues that have precipitated your obesity and be patient. It will take time and patience.

The Victim Mentality

"I have spotted the enemy and the enemy is me!" That familiar quote from Walt Kelly's Pogo cartoon asserts that our challenges and troubles are often complicated by our own perspective. When we remove our ego and self esteem needs, we often find our actions are motivated by needs of approval and acceptance. So many of society's very expensive and pervasive issues are due to our poor self-esteem, lack of knowledge and inconsistent adherence to healthy and productive lifestyles and choices that will ultimately produce the results we desire. Living a healthy, peaceful and prosperous life is simple, achievable and very enjoyable. It is a life built on peace and wellness. Without either, it is difficult to be well adjusted and ultimately prosperous. It requires making the right choices, obedience and focus, A healthy lifestyle plan based on God's word and desires is all you really need, but so many of us have trouble accepting the simplicity of that plan and question our ability to carry it out, but you can with patience and commitment. Don't immerse yourself in your dead past or unborn future. Today is all that matters and when you choose functional health care that is tailored to meet your individual needs and true wellness that includes natural, organic food, alkaline ionic water, healthy supplements, the FIR sauna, adequate rest, fitness (walking, bicycling, swimming, etc), financial prosperity, giving (tithing), healthy relationships and choose love, you will certainly experience peace, joy and prosperity. It is worth whatever changes you have to make and the sacrifices you will endure. Staying focused will get you through the difficult times and the tribulations you may face while letting go of jobs, relationships, homes or people. It is not your fault and your life is all you have. No one can manage your life and the plan for prosperity is unique for your specific needs.

Never think of yourself as a victim. You simply made previous choices that were necessary for that particular time or you are growing and letting go at this time. Put everything in the dead past and unborn future and live only for today. We get one day at a time and that's the way we have to live it – to the best of our ability. Learn to be your best friend who will always support you, forgive you and remind you that you are a child of God, perfect and important. Let go and let the loving Universe support you and love you. You only have your life to live – make it special and do everything necessary to do whatever you feel is important to you. Alone time is often the solution to decide what you value and need the most, not what others think. If you let others live your life for you, that is what they will do. Stand up and move forward. Don't worry about failure or disappointment, they are common to everyone.

Finally, be sure to have succeeding as part of your daily affirmations. You have to "make firm" the process and possibility of success, because it has avoided or eluded you for most, if not all, of your life. Affirmations change your attitude and give you a wonderful ritual to practice everyday to solidify the thought process you need to break the old failure thinking and replace it with positive, optimistic thoughts and goals.

Here is an affirmation I use often. I am radiating and attracting the fruits of the spirit today (love, peace, joy, patience, harmony and prosperity). Also say, "I prosper everyone and everyone prospers me." This affirmation was developed by Catherine Ponder. I read several of her books and I recommend them to you. Joy is for everyone. You have to let go of any cognitive dissonance (stinking thinking) and lead a simple focused, uncomplicated lifestyle that emphasizes living in the "now" and incorporating love, wellness and prosperity in your daily life.

Guilt, anger, worry, depression or the emotional congestion that results from not letting go, seeing yourself as a victim or blaming your unproductive, unhappy life on the complications of 21st century living is wrong and will hold you back from being healthy and happy. You are not a victim or incapable of leading a satisfying life. A great life is a simple life. There are no victims – only victors. It's your choice. Do you choose wellness, love and prosperity or disease, hate and stress?

A Need for Discipline

Discipline is a skill largely unappreciated and virtually ignored by the immature and those who chose to lead a spontaneous and child-like existence. Those who choose to to stay young forever, a lifestyle largely reserved for those of us who live in the richest country in the world, categorically avoid the rigors of life guided by the tenets of discipline. Getting up early, exercising daily, eating healthy whole, organic foods, choosing lifestyle void of all addictions, drinking plenty of alkaline water and seeking adequate rest and sleep are often supplanted by fast food, watching television, driving instead of walking or exercising, popping pills and Doctor visits instead of good nutrition and supplementation and exercising regularly. Americans are basically lazy, undisciplined, stressed and very unhealthy. Our lives are cut short by the lifestyle choices we make. We need a new way of living and we must switch to feel younger, live longer and realize our bodies are capable of living 150 years or more. People in Okinawa are proving that it is possible and it's not genetics, but lifestyle that works for them. They exercise self-discipline with a healthy lifestyle.

It all begins with your attitude. You must be humble, grateful and appreciative. We have to stop believing that people owe us anything. Discipline begins at home. Stop living in denial and embrace progress and healthy change. Let go of the dead past and focus on what your body wants from the neck down, especially. The eyes are interested in how the food looks, the nose how the food smells and the mouth of course, how the food tastes. The rest of your body is only interested in nutrition. You must convert your body to an alkaline pH from an acidic pH and eat only natural foods. Discipline begins at home. Stop being the hare or rabbit and begin to adopt the tortoise or turtle's approach. Take life one day at a time and do what you must do to be successful, healthy and well. Don't complain, take responsibility and stop living in the dead past. Blame is a frequent substitute for discipline. Don't blame anyone but yourself, forgive yourself and move into the moment. Make today a great day.

Follow my program, it worked for me. Don't ever give up. Embrace discipline as a skill, a valuable and necessary skill, to achieve all adult goals such as, marriage, parenting, finances, and wellness. You can be happy and well when you accept and practice disciple on a daily basis. Never resist positive change. Just do it. Expect trials and tribulations and realize that plateaus and unexpected challenges are a very real part of the process and everyone faces those obstacles. Believe in yourself; follow this program and Never Give Up!

Interested or Interesting?

Over 50 years of living on this planet has taught me one very important thing: You can either be an interesting or interested person. It's that simple.

If you choose interesting, as I did for the first part of my adult life, there is often a large debt to pay. Ultimately, most people will grow tired of your self-effacing attitude and no longer seek your company. They will simply tolerate you, if possible. They may also use you, because they know that no one is particularly enamored with you either. You will live an illusion, believing that people respect you and you will feel important, even though you are probably contributing very little, if anything.

In the beginning, they may admire you. Life will appear to be fun and exciting and even wonderful. Every day will seem fulfilling and important to you, until one day you will wake up and realize that your life is empty, misguided and everyone who you thought previously loved you has left you or is using you to meet their needs.

I know the pain and disappointment associated with selfish pride, I understand the empty satisfaction that food, especially sugar, brings. Addiction is a medication employed by humans to cover the pain, depression, anger, anxiety and hurt associated with the complexity, confusion, emptiness and mystery of life. Sometimes, we just do unhealthy things because everyone else does or we simply lack the courage and knowledge to adequately deal with our problems. Denial or delay will only make things worse. You can be more than a conqueror if you take a positive, proactive approach and choose to be interested, instead of interesting.

The people most of us admire: Lincoln, Gandhi, Mother Teresa, Christ and others were all essentially interested people who truly cared about the welfare of others and they knew their needs would always be taken care of. They were satisfied, productive and caring people who gave, sacrificed and make so many people feel better about themselves and that continues today.

You don't have to be a legend, hero or even famous to be happy and prosperous. Be an interested and caring person, but realize that your needs are always covered by your Creator. He is your source for prosperity and success.

Attitude

What does your attitude have to do with prosperity, success or weight loss and wellness? Everything! More than likely a wrong attitude got you to where you are at in the first place. We know the Standard American Diet (SAD) will destroy your life. You can't eat processed food, such as most of the salt, sugar and oils that are sold today in grocery stores are in the foods you eat in restaurants and still expect to feel well and look healthy. By the time you reach your 40's life becomes a downhill journey until the first heart attack, stroke or bout with cancer sends you into a frenzy and worried state of panic.

Your lifestyle and attitude can give you peace, prosperity and happiness. Not only is it important to eat God's food, instead of Man's impure, artificial food loaded with drugs, toxins and impurities, clean your body with natural herbs, detoxify with the FIR sauna, drink alkaline water to rid your body of acidic waste and neutralize free radicals to stop the accelerated aging process. Your healthy attitude of letting go of the problems in your life and seeking the help of your Creator will help you find positive solutions, worry much less and have a positive and optimistic attitude that is possible t lead a long, productive and healthy life. Attitude and lifestyle will get you there.

Your body is designed to live 150 years according to experts at Harvard University.

You just have to neutralize the free radicals, maintain an alkaline pH, hydrate properly, eating plenty of antioxidant foods, cleanse the toxins from your body and be sure it gets the right fuel. It sounds like a lot, but this program is designed to make it easy for you so you can begin to live the clean, energizing and healthy life you want to live. Wellness is truly possible and will happen for you if you stay committed to health. What's the alternative?

Remember, "I have spotted the enemy and the enemy is me!" Take responsibility and follow this program. It will be everything you need to be well and happy.

Time Management

Many Americans often say they lead busy lives, often feel overwhelmed and under supported and basically feel they lead fast-paced lives and are often out of control, even lost. As complicated as daily life can be, the addition of a wellness or weight loss program seems very achievable.

Wellness and weight loss are not nearly as difficult as they might seem if you are organized and follow a few basic steps
1. Eliminate all excuses
2. Always be assertive and consistent
3. Order your priorities
4. Stick to a schedule that works for you
5. Eliminate all superfluous or unimportant things in your life

6. Stick to your plan and schedule
7. You are never to busy – just **unorganized**
8. Practice affirmations on a daily basis
9. Trust yourself
10. Review your plan and schedule – make corrections quickly

Affirmations

I used many affirmations to lift me out of depression, anxiety, and fear and weight loss. They are a way of seeing, believing and knowing what you need to happen will happen. They dissolve the "stinking thinking" so many of us experience every day and turn our negative, failure thoughts into positive optimistic thoughts that guide us and ultimately inspire us to do what we could have done all along. Success begins with "right thinking" and affirmations are the best way to point us in the right direction. You should say them often every day. If you do, your thoughts and mood will begin to change in just a few weeks. You've tried everything else, why not try affirmations and put your whole being into them every day. Success is waiting for you!

Here are a few affirmations I have used:

Daily Affirmations

1. Now is the time of divine completion. The finished results now appear!
2. I radiate and attract joy, love, patience, wellness, harmony and prosperity today.
3. I am living the rich and abundant life God has given me and Jesus died for me to have.
4. I am achieving my highest good today. God's divine love now draws to me all that is needed to make me successful and prosperous.
5. Only success can come into my life. God is watching over me, protecting me from harm and blessing me with overwhelming abundance.
6. I now face the present and future wise, secure and unafraid.
7. I give my treasure, talent and time to help change the world with God's help and guidance.
8. I am trusting God to meet all my needs today. I am successful, confident and free!
9. There is **only** one presence and power in my life: God the good.
10. The Heavenly Father is now helping me to be humble, loving and accepting.
11. I am grateful and deeply thankful for everything God gives me.
12. I am letting go, surrendering to love and dedicating myself to God's will.

13. Today is the only day that matters. I no longer live in the dead past or unborn future
14. The Heavenly Father has forgiven my sins and set me free to love and prosper.
15. By tithing, I am eliminating congestion and gaining circulation.
16. The Heavenly Father is blessing me today. I am prosperous and living a dream.
17. I am attracting abundance and pursuing my passion today.
18. I have an attitude of gratitude and I am deeply thankful for every blessing I receive.
19. The spirit of success is working with me now and I am in all ways guided, prospered and divinely blessed.
20. I call on the great law of restoration. My good of past and present is now divinely restored and pours forth into my life as rich blessings. I joyfully receive and accept them.

www.ingramcontent.com/pod-product-compliance
Lightning Source LLC
Chambersburg PA
CBHW070149290526
45789CB00002B/688